Behind the Eye

By the same author:

Analogue Computing at Ultra-High Speed (with M. E. Fisher). Chapman and Hall, 1962.

Freedom of Action in a Mechanistic Universe. Cambridge University Press, 1965.

The Clockwork Image. InterVarsity Press, 1974.

Science, Chance and Providence. Oxford University Press, 1978.

Human Science and Human Dignity. Hodder and Stoughton, 1979.

Information, Meaning and Mechanism. MIT Press, 1969.

Brains, Machines and Persons. Collins, 1980.

The Open Mind. InterVarsity Press, 1988.

Chapters in:

Man in His Relationships, ed. H. Westmann, Routledge, 1955.

Science in Its Context, ed. J. K. Brierley, Heinemann, 1963.

Man and His Future, ed. G. Wolstenholme, Churchill, 1963.

The Modeling of Mind, ed. K. R. Sayre, University of Notre Dame Press, 1963.

Body and Mind, ed. G. N. A. Vesey, Allen and Unwin, 1964.

Cross Cultural Understanding: Epistemology in Anthropology, eds F. S. C. Northrop and H. Livingston, Harper and Row, 1964.

Readings in Psychology, ed. J. Cohen, Allen and Unwin, 1964.

Cybernetics of the Nervous System, eds N. Wiener and J. P. Schadé, Elsevier, 1965.

Information and Prediction in Science, eds S. Dockx and P. Bernays, Academic Press, 1965.

Christianity in a Mechanistic Universe, ed. D. M. MacKay, InterVarsity Press, 1965.

Brain and Conscious Experience, ed. John C. Eccles, Springer-Verlag, 1966.

Good Reading in Psychology, eds M. S. Gazzaniga and E. P. Lovejoy, Prentice-Hall, 1971.

Non-verbal Communication, ed. R. A. Hinde, Cambridge University Press, 1972.

Handbook of Cognitive Neuroscience, ed. M. S. Gazzaniga, Plenum, 1984.

Objective Knowledge, ed. P. Helm, InterVarsity Press, 1987.

Mindwaves, eds C. Blakemore and S. Greenfield, Basil Blackwell, 1987.

Behind the Eye

Donald MacCrimmon MacKay

The Gifford Lectures delivered in the University of Glasgow
27 October–12 November 1986 under the title

Under our own microscope:
What brain science has to say about human nature

Edited by Valerie MacKay

Basil Blackwell

Copyright © The University of Glasgow 1991

First published 1991

Basil Blackwell Ltd
108 Cowley Road, Oxford, OX4 1JF, UK

Basil Blackwell, Inc.
3 Cambridge Center
Cambridge, Massachusetts 02142, USA

British Library Cataloguing in Publication Data

A CIP catalogue record for this book is available from the British Library.

Library of Congress Cataloging in Publication Data

MacKay, Donald MacCrimmon, 1922–1987:
    Behind the eye / Donald MacCrimmon MacKay; edited by Valerie MacKay
      p. cm.
    'The Gifford lectures delivered in the University of Glasgow,
October–November 1986 with the title Under our own microscope: what brain science has to say about human nature.'
    Includes bibliographical references.
    ISBN 0–631–17332–3
    1. Brain. 2. Neurology. I. MacKay, Valerie. II. Title.
III. Series: Gifford lectures; 1986.
    [DNLM: 1. Brain—physiology—essays. 2. Mental Processes—physiology—essays. WL 300 M1525b]
QP355.2.M33 1990
612.8'2—dc20
DNLM/DLC
    for Library of Congress 90–201
               CIP

Typeset in 11 on 13 pt Granjon by Wyvern Typesetting Ltd, Bristol
Printed in Great Britain by Butler and Tanner Ltd, Frome, Somerset

Contents

Note by the Editor

My husband gave the Gifford lectures upon which this book is based in October and November of 1986. He died in early February 1987 – of the lymphomas with which he had been battling for nearly four years. Thus although the lectures had been taped and were eventually transcribed, only a few pages were edited by him. He asked me to complete the task, working in, where I thought appropriate, material from his other writings, and from the discussions after the lectures with his lively audience in Glasgow. He suggested several friends with expertise in physiology and philosophy who might have the patience to read parts of the manuscript. Wherever work by scientific colleagues is described, I have sent to them the relevant pages for checking. To them and to Dr Neil Spurway (of the University of Glasgow's Gifford lectureship committee), to Drs John M. Forrester, Stuart J. Judge, Oliver Barclay, the Rev. Melvin Tinker and my two sons Robert and David I wish to express my indebtedness and my appreciation.

It is a pleasure to record my thanks also to those who gave permission for their photographic and other visual material to be reproduced and who generously sent me slides and prints of their work.

Knowing that my husband always chose his words with precision, I have preserved as closely as possible the spoken word of the lectures. Apart from inserting about two dozen pages of material from his other writings, I have made only three contributions to the work as now presented: most of the section headings and figure captions and the occasional sentence or paragraph distinguished by the use of italic type in square brackets. References within the text have been kept to a minimum, but there is a bibliography.

Valerie MacKay

About the Author

Donald MacCrimmon MacKay was born in Lybster, Scotland in 1922 and graduated in Natural Philosophy (Physics) at St Andrews University in 1943. After three war years spent on radar development with the British Admiralty he proceeded to research into the ultimate limitations of high-speed electronic analogue computers and into problems of information measurement, receiving his PhD in 1951 for this work.

Having become interested in the differences (rather than resemblances) between computers and the human brain, he spent a year in the USA in 1951 as a Rockefeller Fellow, visiting research workers in neurophysiology and related fields. Thereafter his experimental research was chiefly into the organization of the brain and particularly the information-processing mechanisms of vision, hearing and touch. On the theoretical side he was active from 1946 in the development of information theory (particularly its semantic aspects) and the theory of brain organization, including its philosophical implications.

For 14 years from 1946 he lectured in physics at King's College in the University of London. In 1960 he moved to a new research chair at the University of Keele in Staffordshire. There he built up the internationally known Department of Communication and Neuroscience, in which the resources of physiology, experimental psychology and physics are brought together to elucidate the sensory communication mechanisms of the brain. He became Emeritus in 1982, but continued vigorously in research until a few weeks before his death in February 1987.

He broadcast frequently on radio and TV.

Professor MacKay was one of the founding editors of the international journal *Experimental Brain Research* and of the *Handbook of Sensory Physiology*. He served as chairman of the commission on Communication and Control Processes of the International Union of Pure and Applied Biophysics, and as a council member of the International Brain Research Organization. He was a member of the Physiological Society and of the Experimental Psychology Society, a Fellow of the Institute of Physics, a member of the EEG Society and of the Society for the History and Philosophy of Science, an elected foreign member of the Royal Netherlands Academy of Arts and Sciences and a member of the Neurosciences Research Program of Massachusetts Institute of Technology.

Preface

I will praise thee: for I am fearfully and wonderfully made: Marvellous are thy works: and that my soul knoweth right well.

Psalm 139

The spectacle of our own brain is, of all the structures in the universe, a pre-eminent and proper object of wonder.

Under the provisions of Lord Gifford's bequest, I am required to lecture in 'Natural Theology'. I suppose all forms of speculative theology consider the prime question to be whether the drama or world in which we find ourselves has an Author – and if so, whether that Author has a personal interest in us and claims upon us. Natural Theology I take to mean reflection on such questions in the light of our knowledge of the natural world.

Let me confess at once that I am unhappy about any argument that brings God in as a missing term *within* scientific explanations of the world. There are no facts of brain science known to me that add up to any kind of 'proof' of the existence of God, nor would I expect such a conclusion to follow logically from data of that kind. Science is by its own constitution agnostic. On the other hand there is a real need in our day to bring back a sense of awe into our attitude to the natural world. The invitation is to marvel at the existence of the whole world, the bits whose interconnections we see as well as those we don't understand. This kind of wonder, which no amount of scientific understanding can remove, is quite distinct from and not to be confused with the scientific puzzlement of the exploring scientist which it is his whole ambition to reduce. Nevertheless, there are not a few people in our day, some of them in high academic places, who seem to think that our slowly growing understanding of the mechanisms of the human brain makes it more difficult to take seriously the religious claims that speculative theology would consider to be at least open, and that revealed theology, especially in the Judeo-Christian tradition, would affirm to be sober truth.

I hope, therefore, that Lord Gifford would approve of my devoting these lectures in his memory to a summary sketch of some aspects of brain research with which I have been most closely connected over the past 40 years, interlaced with occasional comments on related philosophical and theological questions regarding our human nature and destiny.

[*Lord Gifford in his will of 1885 expresses the hope that the lectureships which he is establishing will promote 'Natural Theology, . . . the Knowledge of God the Infinite, the All, the First and Only Cause', but desires that they shall do so 'without reference to any supposed special exceptional or so-called miraculous revelation'. This is the background to some of D.M.M.'s remarks above and later.*]

Acknowledgements

Permission to reproduce parts of the text has kindly been granted by the following holders of copyright:

The Controller of Her Majesty's Stationery Office for extracts from 'Operational Aspects of Intellect' in 'Mechanisation of Thought Processes', NPL Symposium No. 10, 1958.

Academic Press, Inc. NY for extracts from 'Recognition and Action' in 'Methodologies of Pattern Recognition', 1969.

MIT Press for extracts from 'Ways of Looking at Perception', in 'Models for the Perception of Speech and Visual Form', ed. Weiant Wathan-Dunn, 1967.

Karger Buchhandlung, Basel for extracts from 'Neurophysiological Aspects of Vision' in 'From Theoretical Physics to Biology', 1973.

1

Under Our Own Microscope

You may think that 12 chapters should give me plenty of time to cover all that needs to be said under the heads I have chosen. But as we shall soon see, the topic of brain science is a vast and rapidly growing one, and in trying to decide what samples to show you and what to leave out I have felt very much in the dilemma of the man whose wife gave him two ties for his birthday. Proudly he came down to breakfast wearing one of them. 'Oh', she said, 'so you didn't like the other one?'

Before we get down to detail, let me try to bring home to you what an exceedingly odd enterprise it is to try to understand our own brain, and what a huge conceptual gap there is between two very different kinds of data which the enterprise requires us somehow to tie together.

Inside and outside aspects

All our psychological functions have what we might call an 'inside' and an 'outside' view. For me, the childhood memory of cycling to school through the chill morning air of the Scottish Highlands is a complex of tingling sensations and vivid mental images. But for you, that memory of mine is inaccessible; what presents itself to you is only an 'outside' view of somebody talking about remembering. My words may, of course, evoke in you some kind of imagined echo of my experience; and you may be able to test some of my descriptions of the past by taking the railway line from Inverness to Bonar Bridge, and then following the road from the manse over the Kyle and up the steep hill behind the village to the school. But however successful this enterprise may be (and I am not sure how good *my* memory is after 50 years) there can be no doubt that you and I have access to radically different aspects of the phenomenon we call 'my remembering'. However well my observable behaviour stands up to your tests, you are not – and cannot be – observing or verifying what I claim to have *experienced* in remembering.

[*Perhaps you might feel that if you could see into my brain while it is working this would bring you closer to what I experience. In some of the chapters that follow we shall indeed try to 'make the head transparent' to see what the brain may be doing during such remembering and experiencing. But we shall find that what we then see is protoplasm and circuitry – an entirely different* kind *of thing from my first-hand experience.*]

The outside view

The picture from the outside is of an ever-active population of some 10,000 million nerve cells or 'neurons', most of which live just under the surface of the so-called 'cortex' or bark of the brain. Practically all our observable behaviour is thought to be determined by the flashing to and fro of electrical impulses among these brain cells, whose interactions govern the timing and intensity of the control signals which are sent out to the muscle system of the body in response to what comes in from the senses. When we learn something new and remember it, the effective pattern of connections between possible paths has been altered. What we should like to tease out are the basic mechanisms upon which the changing state of organization depends. The mechanisms must be quick enough to allow us to absorb some kinds of information at a single glimpse; yet that same information may have to be retained for a lifetime, and it must be readily available in a wide range of relevant contexts.

[*All this and much more can be said, yet still a complete gulf remains – in spite of the points of contact – between this kind of account in terms of nerve cells and electric currents, and my actual first-hand experiencing.*]

The inside view

We can bring it nearer home. If I were to ask *you* at the present moment, 'what are the sort of things you *know* about yourself?', then you might be tempted to tell me stories about what you have read in the literature about the human brain, its molecular constitution, its genetics and so on. That is all very well; these are things you have been told on good authority about your body. But suppose I press you again: 'what are the things you know *most certainly* about yourself?' You might wish to start your list rather differently with indubitable items of the kind: 'I am seeing a room full of people'; 'I feel warm and sleepy'; 'I have a slight toothache'; 'I am trying to think clearly'; 'I like haggis'; 'I believe Glasgow is on the Clyde'; 'I have to decide whether or not to do such and such when I get home', and so on. We could write these in a long column (table 1.1) called the 'I-story', where 'I' stands for inside – and also for I, the first person singular.

Table 1.1   The I-story and the brain-story

Experience *I-story*	*Physical activity* *Brain story*
I feel . . .	Neural activity a
I see . . .	Neural activity b
I hear . . .	Neural activity c
I think . . .	Neural activity d
I like . . .	Neural activity e
I believe . . .	Neural activity f
etc.	etc.

To the left are listed some of the things we know about ourselves 'from the inside'. To the right, the brain scientist assumes that for each entry in the I-story there is a correlate in terms of neural states and events. His working assumption is that no change can take place in our cognitive experience without a correlated change in some neural structure or pattern of neural events in our brain; but the converse is not assumed.

The I-story attempts, in words, to point to data, the immediate, 'given' facts of our conscious experience. These are facts about us. They are *strong* facts in the sense that the data to which these statements bear witness are data we would be lying to deny. We all know how to talk about these because we have learned to share our feelings about our conscious experience, but the data are essentially private. This, I think, ought not to worry us. It has sometimes worried philosophers of science on the ground that it may seem unscientific to base a search for objective knowledge on your own private experience. But when you think about it, this is actually all that any scientist can ever do. He privately either does or does not see the pointer reading 10 on the scale of his recording instrument, and when he writes a paper he has got nothing but that experience to talk about. He may bring in testimony from other observers; but if so, each of them is again only bearing witness to his own private experience. So when we come to study ourselves scientifically, there is nothing to be ashamed of in the fact that one great block of data about ourselves is a block which we must describe in the first person singular. These data are so far from being uncertain or optional that we would be lying if we were to deny them.

Of course, I am not suggesting that when I say 'I see a room full of people,' the fact that the room is full of people is a *fact* that I would be lying to deny. I could be suffering from an optical illusion giving rise to that impression. What I mean is that my *experiencing* seeing-the-room-full-of-people is a fact I would be lying to deny. These are the prime data of our conscious experience – on which even our doubting must be based. All that we know comes in and through *conscious experience* of something or other.

The brain scientist's working assumption

The brain scientist is engaged in trying to supply the second column of table 1.1, which I am going to call the 'brain-story'. His working assumption is that for every fact of experience to which the I-story bears witness there is a corresponding fact about the state of the brain in question. Note that this is only a working hypothesis – there is no solid verification of it – but it is one with good support. [*In later chapters we shall see some of the evidence which points in this direction: evidence from brain-damaged patients, from electrical stimulation of the brain and from recording of the brain's own electrical activity.*]

A major question we are going to be asking is what consequences this working assumption does and does not have for our thinking about ourselves and indeed for the significance of what it is to be human. Our working assumption is that for any change to take place in what you see or hear, what you like or dislike, what you believe or disbelieve, indeed for any change taking place in your conscious experience, some change must take place in the structure inside your head.

On that assumption we are not committed to believing that one and only one brain state corresponds to one fact of your experience. For example, there may be a hundred nerve cells running in parallel so that perhaps any fifty of them, if they fire, will give rise to the same experience. So there is a one-to-many relationship here, but what we are assuming is that no change can take place in your conscious experience without some change taking place in the state or the activity of some part of your brain and nervous system.

Correlated sets of facts

What I want to underline is just how strange this relationship is. Remember we only know any of the entries in the brain-story, or the facts to which they point, through our conscious experience. It is in and through our conscious experience of reading things, looking down microscopes, making measurements and so on that we come to believe that we have a brain at all. All of the brain-story in that sense logically fits inside the I-story as part of what we believe – or at least are prepared to give some credence to. Nevertheless there is this sense in which you can pull out the brain-story from all the mass of other things we believe about the natural world, and lay it alongside the I-story in a kind of correspondence, as we have done in table 1.1. The brain-story entries are not in one to one correspondence with the facts of experience; but we are putting them in *correlation*. We shall spell out, as we go along, more of what that does and doesn't mean. We are assuming that there is a correlate, in the story about your brain, for any fact of your conscious experience and that for any change in the facts to which the I-story bears witness there is a change – a correlated change, we believe – in the brain story.

A science-fiction thought-experiment

Now of course talking in these terms is a discipline which has to be worked through with an eye to possible traps. In order to bring out the sort of thing I mean, I hope you will allow me to introduce one or two simple-minded imaginary thought-experiments. Let us suppose that as you sit in your comfortable chair someone draws your attention to a bench before you, on which there are a number of examinable objects – such as a reading lamp, a radio receiver and the like. Among them let us imagine a brain-like structure immersed in a dish with fluids and a variety of connecting pipes. You are invited to investigate these objects, and let us say that you first of all get some electrical measuring gear and examine the electrical properties of the various objects, the resistances between one point and another, and so on. To begin with all goes well. But when you apply your instruments to the brain-like object in the dish, you have the most extraordinary experience. You suddenly see flashes of light out in space in front of you. You turn the object around and make connections in some of its lower parts and you begin to feel violently sick. What is going on? When you look more closely you find that connected to the foot of this object there is a long cable with a tube carrying blood supply and so on. To your astonishment, you find that the cable actually runs down behind your armchair and in through a socket, fitted by some super-surgeon of the umpteenth century, at the back of your head! What you are looking at, in other words, is your own brain on the end of an extension cord.

All this is, of course, the wildest of science fiction; but I think if we just toy with the idea seriously for a moment it brings out a number of quite interesting philosophical points. There you are, with this connection which we must assume to have been made perfectly so that your experience is just as it would be if the brain were still inside your cranium. In answer to any normal questions, such as 'where are you and what can you see?', you would answer as you always would. You can point to things you can see, you can pick some of them up and you can act as you normally do, sitting in your chair. The fact that your brain is on the end of a cord (we assume) makes no difference.

But now let us ask: when you said just now that you saw flashes of light as you inadvertently poked at this brain-like object in the physical world, where were the flashes of light? It might be tempting to suppose that the flashes of light were located at the place where you poked the brain and interfered with it; but in fact this would not tally with your experience. The perceived location of those flashes of light was actually out in the space in front of you. You could point to them and see them moving about if you moved your eyes,[1] and in various ways locate them there.

So our thought-experiment, trivial though it is, allows us to distinguish two quite different questions. One question is: where is what-

I-am-seeing (where 'what-I-am-seeing' may be, for example, a spot of light)? The answer to that is: it is out in my action-space; it is making a demand on my map of the world in such and such a location. The other question is: where is the physical activity which is the correlate of my experience of 'seeing-the-spot-of-light'? The answer to that is: it is in the brain.

Let us follow it through a bit further. Somebody might say: 'Well, all right, I can now see the trick, there is that cable going round to the back of my head, so that is why, when I poked at the brain out here, I had those weird experiences coming in. Why don't we try interrupting the connecting cable? Of course we must be careful not to cut the blood supply; but suppose we block temporarily the signal lines leading from the brain round behind the chair into my head. What's going to happen?' You might hope that as a result you wouldn't any longer experience those flashes of light when the electrodes were applied to this structure that is out in front of you; but in fact all of our evidence, which we shall be reviewing later, suggests that the contrary is the case. You would go on experiencing those flashes of light, whenever the brain is poked electrically, but you would cease to see the room around you. You would cease to be able to point to things. You wouldn't be able to bear witness to anything more because it is in and through the processing of the information brought from your eyes and your ears via the cable to your brain that you gain the experience of seeing and hearing in the room.

The additional disturbances produced by electrifying your visual brain are additional disturbances to your conscious experience if and only if they bring about changes in the neural activity (called 'b' in table 1.1) which is the correlate of your experience of seeing. So in the brain is where the changes have to occur if you are to have visual experience, even though there is a very important operational sense in which *you* as an agent are sitting in the chair. You are sitting in the chair, the brain is out in front of you, yet disturbances within it give rise to experience which is yours, inescapably, even if the link between your brain and the body in the chair were cut. You see what I mean by saying how odd, how unique – *sui generis* – is the relationship between the vastly complex structure of your brain and your conscious experience.

If you can bear with me, we can dramatize it a stage further. Suppose that the cable is a very long one, on some kind of a reel, and that some tactless individual (having restored the connections so that you do see the world again) puts the jar with your brain in it on a wheelbarrow and wheels it out into the garden so that you see it going down the lawn. Question: where are *you* now? As far as your conscious experience goes you are still sitting in your chair, and you can prove it by telling what is happening in the room, acting in the room, reacting in the room. That is where someone has to come if they want to ask you a question, or want you to pay a bill. You as an agent are still in the chair. But away down at the bottom of the garden, if somebody stimulates your brain, it is activity there that will give rise to your disturbing experiences of nausea or visual hallucinations or whatever. The question 'where are you?' becomes oddly imprecise.

Some philosophical hygiene

You realize of course that I have indulged in this science fiction for a very limited purpose. (Let me hasten to say that since there would be literally billions of connections to be taken care of in such an exercise, I don't expect the science fiction ever to be realized.) I hope it is now clear how very easy it would be in talking of the I-story and the brain-story to overlook a whole minefield of philosophical traps. Questions especially of *where* things are going on, as we shall see, particularly in chapter 5, have to be looked at very closely and scrupulously in order not to make them into nonsense.

One good maxim, I think, is that in an expression such as 'I see-a-spot-of-light-in-front-of-me' or even 'I see-a-room-full-of-people-before-me' it is safest to leave the hyphens in. Seeing-a-room-full-of-people is an experience, one experience. I can break it down by saying whom I see and so forth; but it is an experience which, if I have it, I would be lying to deny. The brain activity that goes on as the correlate of that experience of seeing-the-room-full-of-people may also be some unitary physical activity, and the things you can say about it, including its location, may be categorically different and in general *are* categorically different from the sort of thing you would say about the experience. Hence the value of leaving in the hyphens until you have justification for breaking them up.

What I am pleading for from the outset is that we make a point of observing what you might call semantic hygiene – a determined effort to keep our terms brushed clean of infection by careless confusion of categories. In particular, words like think, believe, hear are words that in their philosophical categories belong expressly to the I-story. It is *people* who think, believe, hear things, like things, see things. Thinking is something people do. The brain-story, we doubt not, has something to be said about it in relation to thinking, such that for any change in what a man thinks, a change must take place in his brain's activity. But to talk about 'brains thinking', I suggest, however common it may be, is philosophically a blunder – a solecism. It is not brains, it is people who think. It is not so much false as nonsense for someone to say 'my brain thinks'. This point is important, of course, when in a later chapter we consider the much debated question of whether machines can think.

This category distinction is one we are going to have to work hard to keep in mind. It would be almost equally a category blunder to say that 'minds think'. There is no ordinary form of speech in which we say 'my mind thinks': we say 'I think'. Talk about mind, as we shall see, stands for a slightly different logical relation.

In saying that 'seeing', 'thinking' and 'believing' are what *I* do, while what happens in my brain is a correlate of this, I do not at all wish to imply that we have to think of the two as parallel streams of different events, maintained in synchronism in some magical way. What I shall be suggesting is that our conscious experience is *embodied in* our brain activity: neither on the one hand identical with it, nor on the other hand quasi-physically interactive with it. Again I am not being dogmatic; this is just a tentative position which we shall be exploring as we proceed. I do, however, believe that there are good grounds at least for denying that the I-story is a mere 'translation' of the brain-story. We shall see later, indeed, that it would be self-contradictory for an agent to believe some of the statements of the brain-story; so they are not translations of his I-story.

In the I-story and the brain-story we are dealing with two groups of facts whose relationship is basically a brute mystery, simply a datum, a given, that we do not understand. It is a 'brute' fact in the sense that there isn't a glimmering of a good reason for it – this fact that, correlated with every change in your experience and mine, there should be a change in the depths of this relatively tiny fraction of the physical world inside your head or mine. I have emphasized, I hope, how weird it is – at least to me – that there should be this connection between the two. The idea that one could say, 'oh, well yes, I see that obviously this is what ought to be going on in the brain if I am experiencing such and such', will, I hope, by the end of this book seem a good deal less plausible than it may now appear. If we can tease out the correlations between them we shall do well. But that there should be such correlations can only leave us wondering.

Looking at our own brains

There is one last preliminary question you might want to ask. (You realize that this chapter is all a kind of prolegomena.) This last question is whether it makes sense to try to understand the brain in all its complexity when we have only got our own brain to do it with. The point of this question is nicely demonstrated if one tries to make a TV camera produce a picture of its own monitor screen. If the camera is pointed elsewhere in the room the monitor screen shows a picture of the chairs and other objects. If, however, we swing the camera to look at its own screen we find it is generating a pseudo picture. And if we zoom in to try and get more detail the whole thing goes haywire. Using a television camera system to look at itself – to get a picture of the picture that it is making – is both technically and philosophically a nonsense. It is on this sort of ground that many people would ask quite seriously whether it can make sense to try to use your brain to understand your brain.

I think it quite clear, and indeed we will come back to this, that this is a technical trap in the way of the brain scientist who wants to use his or her own brain as the object of study, as some of us in fact do. You do have to take precautions to prevent feedback from your measuring or observing device into the brain that is being observed. But for many purposes it is not necessary or even desirable to do the study of brain function on oneself. Generally if one studies the brains of other people or of other animals then there is no feedback of this kind and that kind of objection falls to the ground.

There is of course the problem of scale. As we shall see shortly, we are dealing with a complexity probably greater than the complexity of any other organized structure in the known universe. And therefore indeed our brains are not big enough in a certain technical sense to carry and process all the information we would need from a single brain in order to work out how it functions, even if we knew how to. So, certainly, any hope of developing a brain science in which one knew everything about the brain in the way that a television engineer knows everything about the inside of a TV set must be for ever beyond us. But on the other hand there is nothing to prevent us from abstracting from brain function in the kind of way that, for example, an economist abstracts from the multiple transactions that take place in the world of economics. By systematically refraining from asking questions on a scale that would be beyond us, we can derive general lawful relations, gain an impression of how this acts on that, and in general elaborate a genuine understanding. So it is in this sense, which I think is by no means trivial, that brain science – even the attempt to understand our own brains – is not as senseless as it might otherwise sound.

Notes

1 These statements about the location of percepts are based on experimental evidence such as that described in chapter 5 under 'Electrical stimulation of cortex'.

2

Within the Living Brain

What kind of a structure do we have inside our heads? In this chapter I want to come down to detail and review quickly some of the data we have about the brain – its anatomy and physiology – before returning in chapter 3 to the main question we have been raising as to how brain activity and our conscious experiencing are related.

Plate 1 shows the well-known walnut-like structure of the exterior of the brain with its heavily folded grey outer surface, the cortex. The grey matter contains the bulk of the nerve cell population. Within, if it is sliced apart, is the white matter, the connecting wires of the system. A conspicuous feature, if we approach from above (see plate 2) is the corpus callosum, the great pathway of millions of fibres connecting together the two halves of the 'walnut', the cerebral hemispheres. [*The white matter may do much more than simply connect. The fibre diameters and therefore their conductivities are altered with use and thus are potentially a long term information store.*

Not so conspicuous (see figure 2.1 and plate 2), but far more fundamental and essential to life and the functioning of our whole body are the parts of the brain hidden underneath the cerebral hemispheres and connected both to the spinal cord below and to the hemispheres above. These regions, hypothalamus and brainstem, consist of intimate interminglings of white matter and grey. From them the largely unconscious, partly chemical 'housekeeping' of our bodies is regulated: heart rate, sleep, stomach acidity, water balance, temperature control, breathing, and so on. It is the area of the brain which shows least alteration as we pass from embryo to adult and from lower animals to man.]

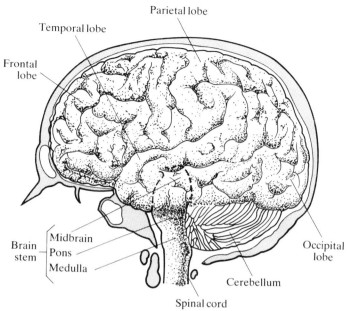

Figure 2.1   Drawing of human brain from left with brain stem and spinal cord sketched in.

The labels on plate 3 indicate the ways in which some of our more conscious activities are associated with the functioning of different regions of the cerebral hemispheres. Vision, for example, is strongly associated with the rear of the brain, speech with the left side and so on. These are intended only as very general indications and you must not get the idea that at the detailed level there is a small scale allocation of function to every brain area. It is possible for people to suffer damage to a good many parts of the brain from bullet wounds or other insults and yet to perform nearly normally. In the young, particularly, the function of the lost or damaged brain areas can to some extent be taken over by neighbouring areas. At any rate the damage to function is not as serious as one might think if one imagined the brain as closely resembling a telephone network or computer. It is true to say, however, that there is a general geographic distribution of functional relationship between different parts of the brain and different aspects of our conscious experience.

The grey matter

Passing to the microscopic level, the individual parts of the brain are remarkably similar in their general structure. In plate 4 we see a slice through part of the folded cortex. It happens to be from the occipital region but would have looked quite similar had it been from almost any part of the cerebral hemispheres. In plate 5 one little corner of a region of the cerebral cortex is greatly magnified and stained. What is immediately clear is that the nerve cell population (of which only a fraction has been stained here) is organized with most of its main connections running radially from the surface. But there is also, as you see, a great deal of lateral connection between the nerve cells.

To put you in the picture for scale, one square millimetre of cortex will have of the order of a hundred thousand nerve cells under it. The strong folding of the cortex enables it to have a total area considerably larger (by a factor of five to six times) than that of the surface of the head. So it has been calculated that we are dealing with a total population of more than 10^{10}: that is to say there are more than ten thousand million nerve cells in each of our brains.

Under the microscope a typical nerve cell looks rather like a minute plant (figure 2.2 and plate 6; for variants see also figure 2.5 and

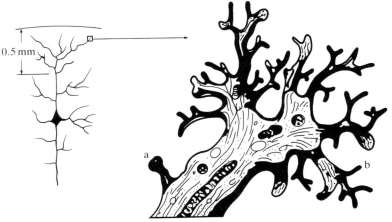

Figure 2.2 On the left is a schematic drawing of a nerve cell; on the right, an enlargement of the area within the tiny square, showing a dendritic tip as drawn from an electron microscope image.

plates 7 and 8). Above the cell body are sensitive incoming dendrites like the twigs or branches of a tree; below it is a long thin tap root called the axon, down which it can send volleys of electrical impulses when it is sufficiently irritated. The axon may extend for many yards on the scale of these pictures and may have collateral branches. [*In figure 2.5 (p. 18) and plates 6–8 the thicker looking, blacker fibres are the dendrites.*]

Under the electron microscope, the interior of the nerve cell in turn reveals enormous complexity (see plate 9), with some of the busiest chemical factories (for their size) in the whole body.

The brain's signalling system

Nerve cells communicate with one another mainly, though not exclusively, by sending a kind of electrical hiccup down the axon. The axon is a fine tube of membrane with different chemicals inside and outside it and you can picture the electric hiccup as something like a smoke ring of electric current which flows between the inside and outside of the tube. It goes down at a speed of from 1 to 120 metres per second, i.e. much more slowly than electric current in a wire. When it reaches the termination at the far end (the synapse, as it is called, which links the cell with another cell) it causes the synapse to spit a minute amount of chemical across the gap. This has the effect of irritating the other cell in such a way as to influence (either positively or negatively) the likelihood that it, in turn, will send out an impulse. So we've got in each of these cells a tiny battery and a means of sending out a smoke ring of current which can provoke activity, or inhibit it, in receiving cells. In general the dead-time between the pulses is much longer than their duration and the pulses emitted by a given cell are all of much the same size, no matter how long or short the intervals between them (see figure 2.3).

The active network

In figure 2.2 a tiny area near the top has been magnified by the electron microscope and shows that the structure is elaborate even on that tiny scale. The labels a and b, for example, mark structures

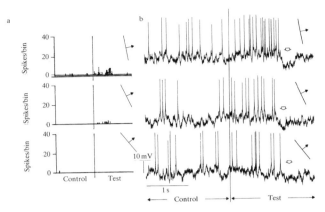

Figure 2.3 Typical trains of pulses, or 'spikes', fired by a cell down its axon. a, extracellular (average of five trials); b, intracellular (single trial) recordings of the responses of the same neurone (complex receptive field) to a moving bar stimulus at the optimal orientations and at orientations 15 and 30 degrees off-optimal (as indicated by bar and arrow). (Martin, 1988.)

called spines. These are believed to be the typical site for a synapse making a link from another cell. These spines are up in the dendrites (they are the bud-like structures along all the dendrites in figure 2.5 and in plates 6–8). The spines may number ten thousand or more on a single cell.

If we continue with our arithmetic, we are thus talking about an organized structure which has 10^{10} times ten thousand, i.e. 10^{14} or a hundred million million, active connections of this or other sorts, any one of which can play a significant part in the overall pattern of activity. So, returning to our thoughts as to the feasibility of using the brain to study the brain, it is clear that one wouldn't live long enough to take in all the data – even if our brains had the capacity to store it – let alone to work out what it all means! We can only work on a sampling basis in trying to understand a system of such complexity.

The synapses in figure 2.4 have been drawn schematically as if, for the most part, they ended on cell bodies. I include this figure because those of you who are interested in computer science will recognize that the synapse landing on a synapse (on the right) forms a special kind of 'gate': it meets the need, common in information-processing circuits, to allow one signal to act as a gate for another without necessarily preventing the recipient element from responding to a third source.

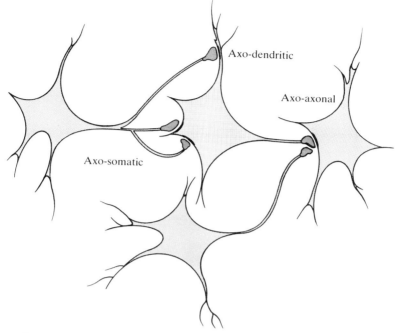

Figure 2.4 Schematic diagram of cell connections.

Signals diffusely distributed 'to whom it may concern' throughout a population of elements might in this way be allowed to reach a selected fraction of the population (MacKay, 1968a).

If you do statistics, however, on *typical* samples, such as plate 5, you will find that a very large proportion (it is now believed the great majority) of synapses in many parts of the cortex are formed not on cell bodies but way out among the dendrites. [*In figure 2.5 the two cells picked out by the staining are making this kind of contact. Plate 9 shows four synapses at high magnification in a section where two axonal fibres happen to be making contact with two spines. The spines are the roughly circular large structures. The synapses are the darker regions indicated by arrows. (The upper axonal fibre is stained black with horseradish peroxidase.)*]

Now this preponderance of contacts out among the dendrites makes a big difference to thinking and theorizing about the brain. Initially, in the late 1940s, there might have been a temptation to say that brain cells (which, as we see in figure 2.3, give sharp pulses of uniform height, with gaps between) do seem a bit like the transistors in a

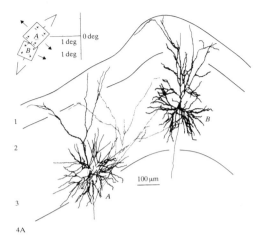

Figure 2.5 Two pyramidal cells. The dendrites are the thicker looking fibres covered in spines. The main axons are the thin fibres descending vertically from each cell body. Some axonal collaterals from cell a make contact with dendrites of cell b. For clarity the complete axonal ramifications of the two cells have not been shown. Horseradish peroxidase stain. Drawing under the microscope by John Anderson. (Martin, 1988.)

computer. In an ordinary digital computer one has transistors that flip from one state into another: either they are 'on' or they are 'off'. So people were inclined in the early days to say, since brains cells too are either firing or not firing, that perhaps if we do enough theorizing about digital computers we shall come up with theorems that will apply to the working of the brain. But in fact the dendrites of typical nerve cells branch in an immensely complex way, as plates 6–8 make clear. The presence of an irritation at one point can give rise to spreading activity in dendrites which, in its turn, can have a highly complex action on the signals from hundreds or even thousands of other synapses. You see the point: that if you've got a large sensitive branchwork at the top of your tree and if irritation of one twig can cause, as it were, electrical or chemical shivers to run through the whole branch, then the responsiveness of that branch, and of any other part affected by it, to other input is going to be changed.

I mention these technicalities as pointers, not so much to sheer complexity, as to the *kind* of complexity that we are going to have to take for granted in thinking about brain function. We are not thinking of something that has the clickety-click easy formalizability of a digital computer where everything is either 'on' or 'off' and one can write formulae with ones and zeros to represent the state. We are talking about a structure whose physico-chemical state can vary smoothly from one state to another, suffer small virtually continuous changes in excitability as a result of signals converging from hundreds or thousands of other fibres. And we are dealing with the net effect of interaction of 10^{10} of such elements with all this complexity of interlacing between the elements themselves.

We are going to have to be content – indeed some would say it is a liberation! – to make do with statistical conceptions of the way that the brain functions and not rush happily to analogies with digital computer programs (see MacKay, 1960b).

Why are nerve connections so 'random'?

Figure 2.6 shows a sample of the tangle of connections between cells under only 1 mm of the visual cortex of the cat – and this with only 1 per cent of the nerve cells revealed by the staining. I show it because you might begin by saying 'this is just a random mess', and then, 'maybe this is another statistical aspect of the brain; that it can only grow in a mess and perhaps statistically organize itself as time goes on'. Now there is a good deal of evidence that the brain does change its organization as time goes on, but I think it is important for us not to imagine that this is for lack of nature's ability to wire it up neatly if there is a need.

Orders of magnitude are difficult to be sure about, but it has been computed that there is not enough information available in the genetic code of man to detail the wiring of every cell in the brain to every other. So in that sense there has to be, if not randomness, at least a good deal of redundancy in the way the system is wired up by nature. And this is all to the good because learning and other things are believed to depend upon the alterability, if not of connections, at least of the *strengths* of connections by, for example, thickening or thinning the necks of those dendritic spines that we were looking at in figure 2.2.

To see that nature is capable of specifying wiring rather neatly, consider plate 10. This is a photograph from the work of Dr Valentino

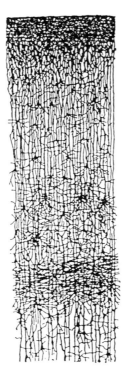

Figure 2.6   Typical sample of intercell connections in the cerebral cortex.

Braitenberg on the visual network of the fly. The house fly has a beautifully regular mosaic of optically sensitive elements in its eye and behind them there lies this wonderfully regular, highly repetitive, lattice of interconnections. So when nature, metaphorically speaking, needs to do things neatly, she evidently can.

The same point is made by plate 11, which shows the receptor cells in a fly's eye. You notice that the groups of cells all have the same orientation above the midline of the photograph, and then below it there is a reversal of the sort that you sometimes come across in crystals. When the biological machinery needs to grow things with crystalline regularity it evidently can do so not merely at the molecular level but even at the level of such highly organized entire structures as the photosensitive cells of the eye.

The appearance of randomness that we noticed in figure 2.6 probably has to do with the fact, to which we shall return later in this chapter, that if a system dealing with the visual world is to be able to cope with all the rich variety that it will come across in that world, it is a positive advantage not to build in too strong a prejudice in favour of one pattern rather than another. [*Plate 8 shows the structuredness occasionally found within the apparent 'tangle' of the cat's brain. The axonal branchings in this plate are the most regularly spaced ever seen in a mammal.*]

The need for good questions

So here we are, looking at a system with 10^{14} active elements and we must think of it as not just sitting there waiting for something to happen, but as engaged most of the time in some kind of cooperative dance. If you record electrical activity from the brain of a human being or other animal you find that many of the nerve cells are active even in sleep, and although others are quiet and waiting for input, the system as a whole tends to lock into cooperative patterns somewhere or other at any given time. The same Dr Braitenberg has humorously described a human life as just a matter of 10^{10} impulses rushing over 10^{14} synapses!

How are we going to make sense of all this? Looking at the anatomy seems rather discouraging. What we need is not more anatomical information, although that is valuable. What we need are good questions to ask about the tangle that neuroanatomy puts before us. There has been a great deal of progress in tracing individual nerve fibres over long distances by injecting, for example, horseradish peroxidase (as in plates 6, 7 and 8). This chemical tends to spread along the fibres from a cell, making it possible to trace a fibre from, for example, the base of the brain right up into the cortex. Neuroanatomical knowledge is thus growing rapidly as to where individual cells come and go, but what we badly need is more ideas about what kinds of questions to ask of the data.

By way of an example of one idea that may be hopeful, consider the two diagrams in figures 2.7 and 2.8. Figure 2.7 is a learning mechanism designed by engineers. It is a network which is able to look for statistical connections between inputs that are arriving in parallel, in such a way as to learn for itself what it is, say, about a speech sound that makes it recognizable by human beings as the vowel 'ah' or 'ee' or whatever. It does this by having all these parallel inputs connect

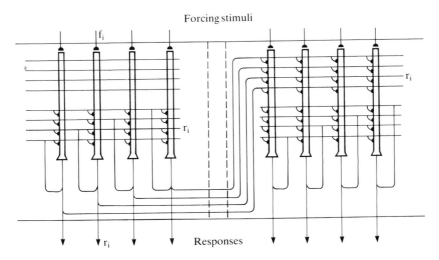

Figure 2.7   An associative network designed to 'learn' and respond to patterns (in speech sounds). Elements, f_i, of the forcing or afferent stimulus pattern are fed in at the top. Elements, r_i, of the response pattern are fed back into the network at shorter and longer distances. The vertical dotted lines separate the two subsystems shown, and the horizontal solid lines represent the surfaces of the laminar network. (Kohonen et al., 1981.)

through adjustable connections (rather like the synapses we have been talking about) on to elements which add up the total 'weight' of the information coming in. This weight is a kind of product of the strength of the activity and the strength of the connection in each case. By modifying these connections in obedience to feedback from the human being who is training the mechanism to recognize the pattern in the sound or whatever, the device, after enough training, can print out of its own accord the appropriate phoneme in response to a particular sound.

Figure 2.8 is a diagram produced by neuroanatomists and neurophysiologists studying a particular part of the brain (concerned, in fact, with the sense of smell). There are parallel connections and upward collectors and a kind of recurrent feedback: altogether you see there are quite striking resemblances with figure 2.7. I show this not, of course, to say that the theoretical model of Kohonen explains how this anatomy works, but to show what I mean by needing good questions. What the engineers have suggested is a possible role for the

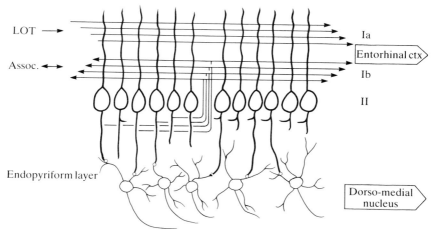

Figure 2.8 A diagrammatic summary of some of the major features of the organization of the pyriform layer (based largely on the work of Price and Slotnick, 1983). The lateral olfactory tract (LOT) enters an array of dendrites and forms an extensive terminal field in layer Ia. The dendrites belong to a layer of neurons whose cell bodies form layer II and whose axons collateralize in layer Ib as a dense associational projection (Assoc.), and send branches into the endopyriform nucleus, i.e. the deep layer of the pyriform cortex. (The similarity between the form of the circuitry in figures 2.7 and 2.8 was pointed out by G. Lynch, 1986.)

anatomical circuitry: they have provided the anatomists with a set of questions they might not otherwise have thought of asking. Is this piece of tissue, for example, picking out particular patterns in the incoming flux of signals?

Now it is a weary business going through questions, with nature giving you the answer 'no' to one after another. It is quite likely that you start off with what sounds like a good question and nature simply says: 'No, that is not what I am doing at all. I have quite a different principle in mind.' But that is the way it has to go if we are to make sense of anatomical data.

Neurophysiology: single cell recording

Another way of piecing together what goes on in the brain has been the very widely exploited development of recording from single nerve cells.

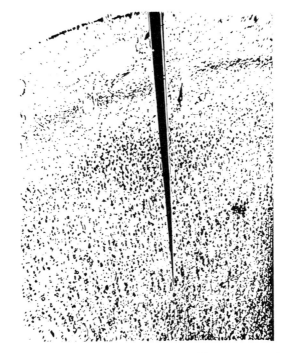

Figure 2.9   Slice from auditory cortex of cat with tungsten microelectrode on same scale. The thickness of the grey matter is about 2 mm. The stain is cresyl violet, which stains only the cell bodies. (Evans, 1964.)

Figure 2.9 shows a little slice of the auditory cortex of the cat and on the same scale a microelectrode. This is a very fine tapered insulated tungsten wire or glass pipette pulled to a diameter of a few millionths of a metre so that its tip is small compared with most nerve cell bodies. If a glass tube is used, it is filled with conducting fluid. When the electrode comes close to (or touches) a cell body, it is possible, by amplifying the current that is picked up through the metal or fluid of the electrode, actually to listen to individual nerve cells firing off. Played over a loudspeaker the sound is rather like machine gun fire at a rate of a few tens or hundreds per second. What one is overhearing is the hiccups or smoke rings which we talked about earlier. [*The records in figure 2.3 were obtained using microelectrode techniques.*]

Using such a device, it has been discovered that some cells in the brain are specifically sensitive to sounds of a particular frequency. The experimenters play a random sequence of tones to the anaesthetized animal and to just one frequency the cell responds with a brief rattle of firing. In the case of another type of cell, Evans (in 1964) found that when he played a gliding tone, sweeping up or down the scale, some cells responded only to the rising or falling sweep but not to any other input. So in various ways it is possible to label individual nerve cells in the cortex with what is called their 'preferred feature'.

Now many cells, as we shall see, have *more than one* preferred feature so it is not at all as simple as just discovering a kind of written alphabet in the brain where every nerve cell has its alphabetic tag attached to it. Cells very often have to cooperate, perhaps communities of thousands of them together, to do the kind of analytic job that is needed when one particular sound has to be recognized. Nevertheless, this general approach of microelectrode recording from single cells has proved one of the most fruitful ways of making sense of what otherwise is a baffling complexity.

Just as in the auditory system there are cells which have, so to speak, a preference, a responding preference, for particular sounds, so in the visual system also there are cells which are not vigorously active until very particular visual stimuli are presented in their own particular region of the visual field. Hubel and Wiesel were awarded the Nobel prize for their work from 1959 onwards, revealing that in the visual cortex there are many cells which are sharply sensitive to the orientation of such things as a black bar or a bright bar on a neutral background. If the bar is swept to and fro at one angle in front of the eye of the anaesthetized animal the cell will respond, but if the bar and its direction of sweep are turned through a right angle the cell ceases to respond. Systematic exploration has shown that all possible orientations of black–white edges are, in this sense, represented in the cell population.

Cells are feature sensitive rather than 'feature detectors'

There has been a school of thought among neurophysiologists, following these discoveries, that each cell was like a letter of the alphabet signalling the presence of one feature. The physiological notion of 'feature detection' came to prominence in the classic paper by Lettvin et al. in 1959 on 'What the frog's eye tells the frog's brain'. Their suggestion had been that a visual cell showing centre–surround antagonism[1] could be thought of as signalling the presence of a small object against a contrasting background and so could serve as a 'fly detector'.

When Hubel and Wiesel in 1959 reported the sensitivity of their 'simple' and 'complex' cells to the orientation of edges or bars of luminance contrast, it seemed natural to dub these cells 'edge or bar detectors'. It seemed attractive to think of such cells as performing the first steps towards pattern recognition by analysing the retinal image into an array of oriented line elements. Theories of global pattern recognition were advanced, involving a kind of analytic hierarchy for extracting pattern invariants and built in its lowest tiers upon the 'simple' and 'complex' cells, some of whose specificities were known. At the apex of the hierarchy there would be a population of 'grandmother cells', whose firing would signify the presence of specific Gestalts such as grandmother's face (or whatever) before the eye. It is no longer fashionable to take this seriously.

Implicit in such thinking was the idea that every cell had one private label, so that when it fired you could guarantee that that particular feature was present. In fact, however, my colleague, Peter Hammond, and I discovered that there is one whole class of Hubel–Wiesel cells (the 'complex' cells) which are sensitive not merely to sweeping by bars of light, but also to the 'brushing' of their region of the retina with a random speckle texture of the general kind shown in figure 2.10. That is to say, *either* of two dissimilar stimuli causes these cells to fire.

Our reason for making the experiment in the first place was to discover whether the Hubel–Wiesel cells were sensitive to something that all of *us* are sensitive to. All of us are sensitive to bar shapes in general; not only to black ones on white backgrounds but also to bars defined by contrast of texture or by motion of texture. For example, if you cut a strip of static noise and move it over a background of similar texture it is clearly recognizable as to its shape and its movement – so long as it moves. But if it stops moving it disappears, it melts back into the camouflage – like a leopard in the bush. Our question was, do Hubel–Wiesel cells respond to that sort of stimulus?

The answer turned out to be that ordinary 'simple' Hubel–Wiesel cells, which are sensitive to a black or a white bar or edge, are not

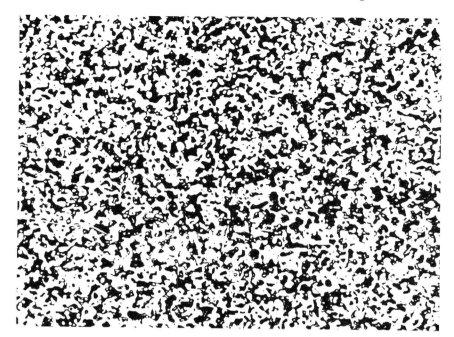

Figure 2.10   Random texture, also referred to as 'static visual noise'.

sensitive to such movement; but the 'complex' cells are sensitive. On the other hand, they do *not* care about the orientation or the shape! If you wave a whole card of visual noise in front of the eye of the anaesthetized animal, you will find that complex cells tend to respond to movement regardless of the shape of the edges of the card. Moreover they respond to movement of the fine random speckle in directions other than the direction in which they prefer a black or white bar to move!

Thus the same 'complex' cell may respond in a highly specific fashion both when confronted with a white bar moving with one orientation and direction of motion, *and* when confronted with random noise moving in one or more other directions. This rules out the otherwise attractively simple idea that each cell in the visual brain is 'labelled' with one particular feature to which it is sensitive, so that its firing *signifies* the presence of that feature.

Nevertheless, there is a very encouraging system and order about this kind of specific sensitivity shown by different cortical cells to particular features of the sensory field.

Studies of cell populations

[The above studies, both anatomical and physiological, have focused on the individual cell. Let us now stand back a little and see what larger groups of cells are doing en masse.]

Hubel and Wiesel have used a technique of autoradiography to trace the connections from the eyes right through to the striate cortex. One eye was injected with a substance, proline-fucose, which is slowly transported along the nerves. A few of the hydrogen atoms in this substance had been replaced by their radioactive isotope tritium, so two weeks later, when the brain was sectioned, those regions reached by the radioactive marker showed up under the microscope. The result is the beautiful arrangement within layer IVc shown in plate 12. Some 50 bands of cells connected to the injected eye show up white on the plate. They are arranged in alternating fashion with dark bands from the other eye. [*The bands are about the width of the lines of one's fingerprint. Indeed when photographed in the plane parallel to the surface of the cortex, i.e. perpendicular to the plane of plate 12, they look not unlike fingerprints.*]

A similar picture has emerged using the elegant technique of Dr Louis Sokoloff. This is based on the amount of *work* being done – how 'hungry' the cells are – within these left and right eye bands. A glucose-like molecule containing a radioactive label is fed into the bloodstream while one eye of the animal is covered and the other is in use. In both halves of the cortex those bands of cells which are more vigorously active while the deoxyglucose is around take up more fuel and so become marked with the radioactive label. These kinds of technique have enormously increased our understanding of that tangled felt-work that we looked at in figure 2.5 and plate 5.

One of the most exciting developments of the past few years has been made possible through the discovery of certain dyes which can be used to mark neurons in the *living* animal. These change their optical fluorescence according to the voltage field in which they lie. For example, if neurons in a particular place are hyperpolarized then the dye will emit more light; if they are relatively more depolarized it will emit less. With this technique it is possible to look down a microscope (with a TV camera and suitable electronics) and record the shifting pattern of light and shade over the cortex of the anaesthetized animal while its eyes are being fed visual diets of different sorts.

Plate 13, for example, shows four pictures from the same 8 mm wide patch of cortex. In the lower two pictures you can see dark patches indicating sensitivity to one orientation of a bar, separated by contrasting patches which indicate lack of sensitivity to that orientation. Here is direct evidence of a segmentation of regions of the cortex within a millimetre of one another, according to which orientation of stimulus they prefer. In the upper right-hand photograph you have the bands, which we talked about in connection with plate 12, corresponding to stimulation of one eye as against the other.

I mention all this to give a feeling for the sense in which we are closing in on the *current* activity of the brain. We are becoming more and more able to visualize and actually to study, through the microscope, the dance of activity in the living brain at the moment of activity, instead of having to wait for hours or days to get our picture.

Computation and cooperativity

The above techniques of making activity visible describe not so much the individual cells as groups of cells. It should be emphasized that when we say that 'a particular cell is sensitive', our statement is based on sampling, and we may, for all we know, have picked up one member of a *team* of a hundred or more, and perhaps if it were not for the whole hundred, no cells would be specifically sensitive. But with that caveat, let me say that other workers, notably Professor Zeki of University College London, have recently been able to identify a whole succession of sub-areas of the visual cortex of the cat and the monkey in which most of the cells show a preferred sensitivity; in one area to colour, in another to movement in particular directions, regardless of what is moving, and so on.

So these tangles of connections between cells, which at first look as if they are a mess and must be blurring the visual picture, ought perhaps to be thought of as more like the tangle of wires at the back of a computer. Not that the brain is a digital computer, but the nerve cells are interactive with one another so as to perform computations on the figure of excitation landing on the retina. Different regions of the cortex perform different classes of computation, one class bringing out particularly the orientation of lines, another bringing out the texture, another bringing out the motion, another the colour and so on.

These grouped activities resulting in sensitivity in single cells are a special case of phenomena which go by the general name of cooperativity, and which are very common in the nervous system. When you think about it, all these cells are little batteries and little amplifiers, and as any one knows who has tried to use an amplifier in a situation where the microphone gets too near the loudspeaker, it is much more likely than not that, unless you take special precautions, a system like that will indulge in cooperative activity. It may 'howl' in the way that we often hear microphones doing when they are mal-adjusted, or alternatively, perhaps, dance in a particular pattern, flipping from one dance to a different one as voltages, connectivities or other conditions are subtly changed. Cooperativity is very common in large groups of cells and the brain is well organized to prevent this sort of cooperativity normally from getting out of hand. (Epileptic seizures are one form of disorder in which the cooperativity does get out of hand, and the cells run amok exciting one another, presumably in somewhat the chaotic way in which a loudspeaker can excite a microphone.)

[*A more technical paragraph to similar effect follows (from MacKay, 1960b, 1980b).*]

The general idea of distributive information-processing goes back at least to Lashley in the 1920s and 1930s. My purpose is not so much to press this as a hypothesis as to keep alternatives alive in our minds at this early stage of the game. What I am suggesting is that we should carry our statistical model-making to the point where the entities we treat are not the electrical or physical elements but patterns or waves of their activity, with laws of motion and interaction of their own – relatively free to move through the neural substrate, much as ripples can move over the surface of a pool, or flames flicker over a coal fire. We must not ignore the possibility that biological recognition of different patterns may require only the existence of what a physicist would call mutually exclusive 'Eigenstates', stable modes of coupled activity involving a fair proportion of the neural population. This is not to deny (what we already know) that specific units may be silent unless specific features are present; it means only that their activity may contribute to the moulding of transition-probabilities between dynamically active states of a large population as a whole, rather than by setting the threshold of a single final unit.

Large scale recording with good time resolution

In addition to studying single cells or tiny areas of cortex it is therefore valuable to have means of studying the *mass* activity of relatively large areas of cells. If you like an analogy, it can give you sometimes the sort of information that you can derive about weather prospects from the satellite cloud map for Europe but would have found hard to deduce from looking at the clouds overhead in one locality.

Electrical – the electroencephalogram (EEG)

This is a technique which goes back quite a few years (to Berger 1929; Adrian and Matthews, 1934) but is still being elaborated. Figures 2.11 and 2.12 relate to one form of the method from our work at Keele. What we do is to apply electrodes as in the ordinary hospital EEG, but we apply them in a regular pattern of the sort you see in the alternative examples of figure 2.11. For any of the ringed electrodes there are three neighbouring electrodes in a symmetrical arrange-ment. If, from the signal at the middle electrode, we subtract the

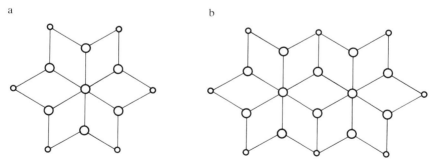

Figure 2.11 Electrode layouts for (a) seven and (b) twelve channel arrays. The large circles denote the 'Laplacean' channels. Each of these is sur-rounded by three neighbouring electrodes whose voltage is averaged and subtracted from that of the centre electrode to obtain (an approximation to) the current source-density. (MacKay, 1983; MacKay et al., 1986.)

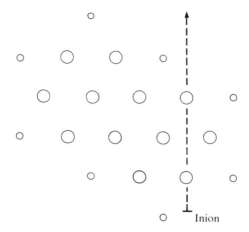

Figure 2.12   Electrode array used to obtain, for the locations represented by large circles, the results shown in figure 2.13. The array was at the rear of head as shown in plate 14. The dotted line represents the midline of the back of head from the inion up towards the vertex. Electrode spacings 1.5 cm. (MacKay, 1984.)

average of the potentials at its three neighbours, we are performing a rough mathematical approximation to the curvature of the potential. If you wonder why one should bother, think of children in the garden under a little tent. Of course their little heads are pushing around on the sloping roof of the tent and where there is a curvature, a bulge, you know there is a child. If you want to know where they are, you follow the bulges. In just the same way, if there is a generator of potential in the head, a source of electric field on the scalp, arising in the brain, one way of identifying it and seeing it move around is to look out for the bulges in the electric potential field over the scalp. This method allows us to do it, in this case in a dozen locations simultaneously.

[*The following experiment puts the method through its paces. The mapping of part of the subject's visual field onto the occipital region at the rear of his head is explored.*]

The subject is fixating a point towards the upper left corner of a television screen (as indicated in the small diagram at the top left of figure 2.13), while the little $\frac{1}{2}$ degree diameter pattern (shown enlarged at the top of figure 2.13) is presented in random order at

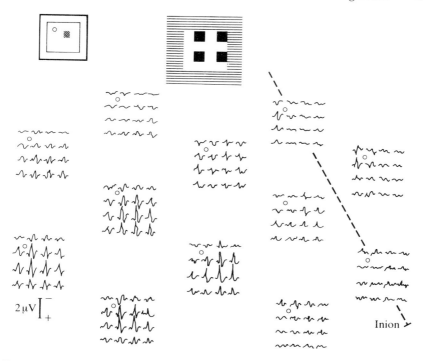

Figure 2.13 Receptive field plots in occipital region (see plate 14) for the 12 scalp locations represented by large circles in figure 2.12. The dotted line represents the midline of the back of the head. The voltage swings are recorded simultaneously at each of the 12 scalp locations for 243 ms following the onset of the checked pattern (inset top right) at any one of 16 possible positions near the point of fixation on the screen (inset top left). The fixation point is represented by O in each case. For every trace 256 graphs are averaged. (MacKay, 1984.)

each of 16 positions on the screen (mostly to the right of and below the fixation point). A computer adds up the electrical responses at each of 12 locations on the head to the presentation of that little pattern in each of the 16 positions. So you get a kind of map. The most conspicuous feature of this particular map is that the electrodes at the lower left of figure 2.12 (which were about 5 cm to the left of the middle of the back of the head) show strong sensitivity to movements of the little pattern over a region of the visual field about 2 degrees in diameter, below and to the right of the centre of gaze. Just $1\frac{1}{2}$ cm away the next scalp electrode shows practically no sensitivity.

The take-home message is that using this kind of technique one can get spatial resolution (i.e. the ability to separate what different regions of the underlying brain are doing) of the order of 1 cm even though one is recording right through the scalp and the bones of the skull. This is an encouraging step towards mapping brain activity and we shall see more of it in later chapters.

[In passing we notice that the part of the brain to the left *of the midline is responding to the visual field to the* right *of the fixation point. This crossing over, whereby the right of the outside world is represented in the left half of the brain, and the left half of the world in the right cerebral hemisphere, is a general feature of brain architecture which we shall meet again.]*

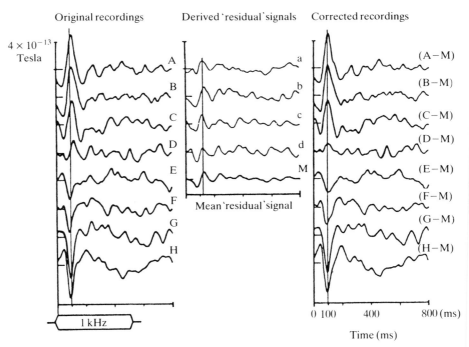

Figure 2.14 Magnetic fields from the right side of the head in one subject in response to a 1 kHz stimulation of the contralateral ear (60 responses averaged). The locations A (posterior) to H (anterior) are spaced at intervals of 7.5 mm and extend to both sides of the Sylvian fissure. Upward deflections indicate a magnetic field direction into the head. (Elberling et al., 1982; reproduced with permission.)

Magnetic field recording

In figure 2.14 we have a sample of a newer method of large-scale recording where what is recorded is the *magnetic* field generated by groups of brain cells. This particular recording comes from the auditory region in a human subject. You will notice that even in the uncorrected original recordings, to the left of the figure, this method of recording the magnetic field at the surface of the head (generated by the tiny currents going through the neural population underneath), gives rather clean signals in response to a 1 kHz tone peep. In order to obtain this kind of sensitivity to magnetic fields one has to use superconducting quantum-interference devices, known for short as 'SQUIDs'. This means using liquid helium, apparatus with a structure that is non-magnetic, and doing the experiments after local electrical equipment has stopped for the night. Nevertheless, it can be used as an alternative to sticking electrodes on and can sometimes do better in picking up signals from the depths of the brain.

There are other large scale techniques using blood flow which we shall be coming to later (in chapter 6). [*They have the merit of locating all activity within any given two-dimensional slice through the head, but the time resolution they currently offer is of the order of a second.*]

Summary

The great complex tangle of cells inside our heads can be made to reveal some of the things it is doing, including some of the functionally significant things it is doing using methods of recording from single cells and also using what one might describe as 'weather map' studies of the electrical and magnetic gross potentials which can be picked up from outside the human head.

[*The above illustrations happen all to be concerned with the brain as a receiver of inputs – largely because many of the most beautiful discoveries of the past 20 years have been on the sensory side, both visual and auditory. This choice of illustrations may thus convey the misleading impression that all the brain has to do is to function rather like a television camera, filtering, analysing and generally processing the incoming signals in such a way as to produce a sharp reconstituted image of the external world on some 'neural screen' inside the head. But of course any animal is much more than a passive receiver of sensory inputs. The frog flicks out its tongue and catches the passing fly. The dog pricks its ears and becomes ready to welcome or repel on hearing a step at the gate. Thus sensory input leads (typically) to action; it shapes the course of present and often of future action. And the activity will be not just any action, but activity which serves the animal's interests. So in the next chapter we turn our attention to agency, that is to activity, both internal and external, in view of ends. When we later return to the topics of learning and perception it will be from this perspective of the organism as a functioning whole.]*

Notes

1 A cell is described as showing centre–surround antagonism when its response to the presentation of a stimulus (for example, a small dark patch in a particular region of the visual field) is enhanced by the addition to the stimulus of a contrasting surrounding zone.

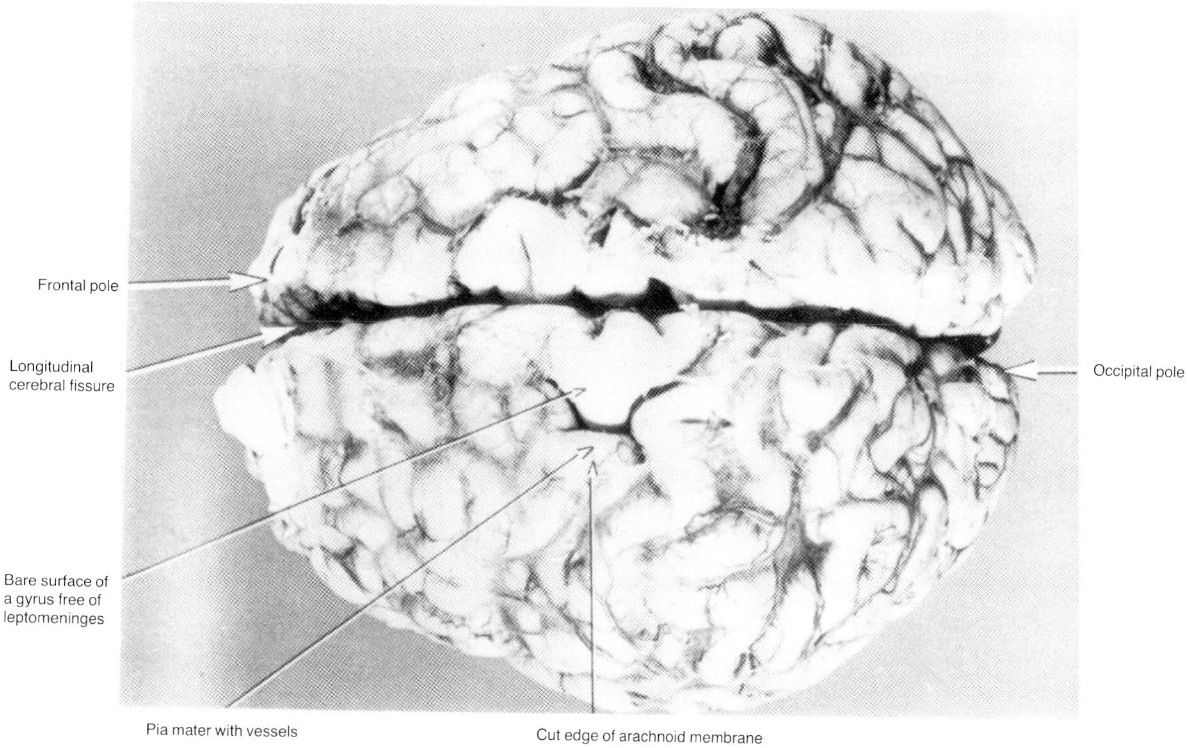

Frontal pole

Longitudinal cerebral fissure

Bare surface of a gyrus free of leptomeninges

Occipital pole

Cut edge of arachnoid membrane

Pia mater with vessels

Plate 1 Human brain viewed from above. The occipital region is at the rear of the head. (Ford et al., 1978.)

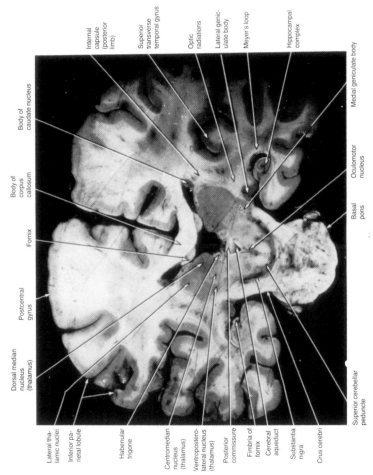

Dorsal median nucleus (thalamus)

Body of caudate nucleus

Body of corpus callosum

Fornix

Postcentral gyrus

Internal capsule (posterior limb)

Superior transverse temporal gyrus

Optic radiations

Lateral geniculate body

Meyer's loop

Hippocampal complex

Lateral thalamic nuclei

Inferior parietal lobule

Habenular trigone

Centromedian nucleus (thalamus)

Ventroposterolateral nucleus (thalamus)

Posterior commissure

Fimbria of fornix

Cerebral aqueduct

Substantia nigra

Crus cerebri

Superior cerebellar peduncle

Basal pons

Oculomotor nucleus

Medial geniculate body

Plate 2 Vertical section through the brain and brain stem (pons). Note the deep folding of the cortex, and the corpus callosum connecting the two hemispheres. (Ford et al., 1978.)

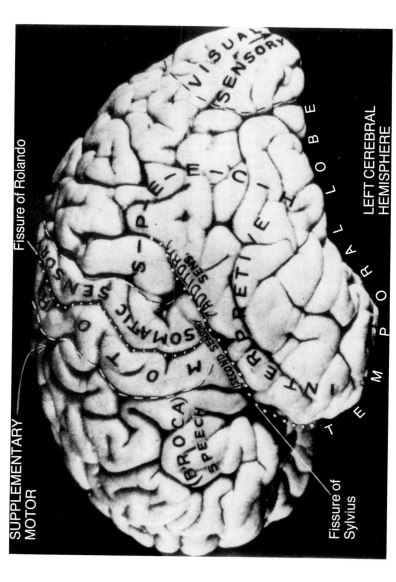

Plate 3 Left cerebral hemisphere showing areas devoted to speech, sensation and voluntary movement. The region of cortex at which electrical stimulation produces experiential 'flashbacks' lies within the area labelled 'interpretive'. (Penfield and Roberts, 1959; copyright © 1959 Princeton University Press, reprinted by permission of Princeton University Press.)

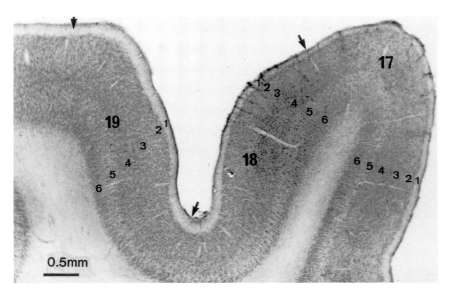

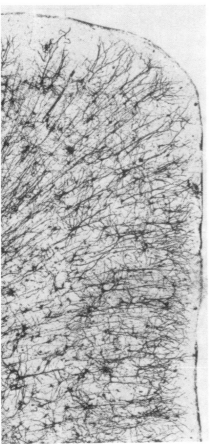

Plate 4 (above) Microscope section of part of visual cortex of the cat (Nissl stain). The same six-layered general structure is found in all cortical areas. (Martin, 1988.)

Plate 5 (left) Microscope section of sensori-motor cortex in cat. The nerve cells are stained by the Golgi method which makes visible about 1.5 per cent of the cells present. (Sholl, 1956.)

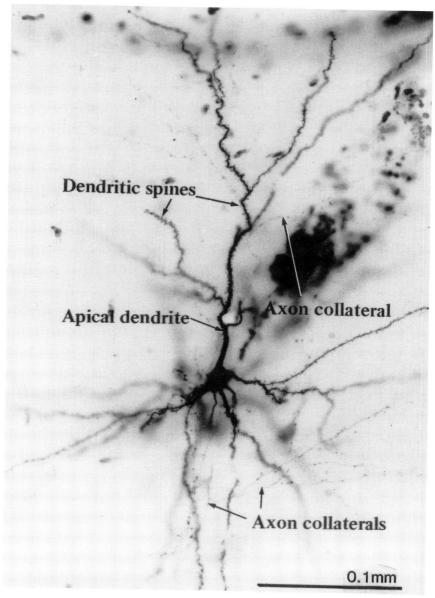

Dendritic spines

Apical dendrite

Axon collateral

Axon collaterals

0.1mm

Plate 6 Photograph of a typical cortical cell (a pyramidal cell) stained with horseradish peroxidase. The main axon is the thin vertical fibre below the cell body. (Martin and Whitteridge, 1984.)

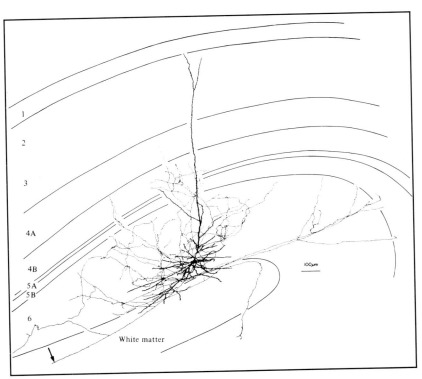

Plate 7　A pyramidal cell of layer 6. Drawing under the microscope by John Anderson. The main axon (arrowed) projected to another region of the brain. (Martin, 1988.)

Plate 8　A spiny stellate cell of layer 4A. The axon formed bouton clusters (arrowed) spaced approximately 1 mm apart. (Martin and Whitteridge, 1984.)

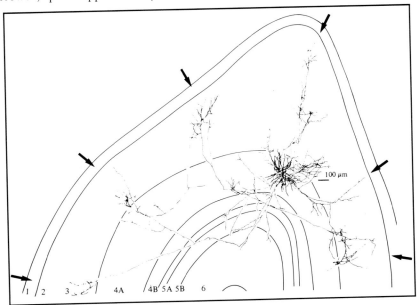

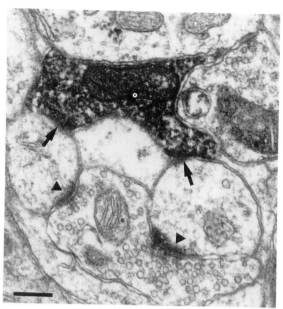

Plate 9 Electron microscope photograph of section through two spines which are receiving synapses (arrowed regions) from two axonal fibres. The upper axonal fibre is black, being filled with HRP stain. It is thought to come from an inhibitory cell, whereas the other axonal bouton is thought to come from an excitatory cell; hence the difference in the synapses. Such dual inputs (excitatory and inhibitory) are thought to occur on only 7 per cent of spines. The bar is 0.2 μm long. (Somogyi et al., 1983.)

Plate 10 Network of nerves connecting ommatidia in housefly. (Braitenberg, 1977.)

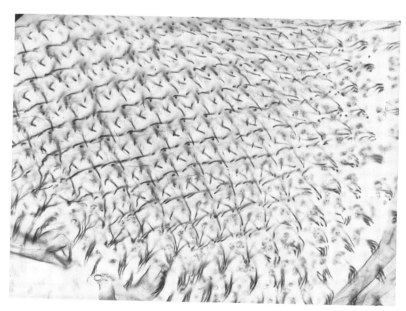

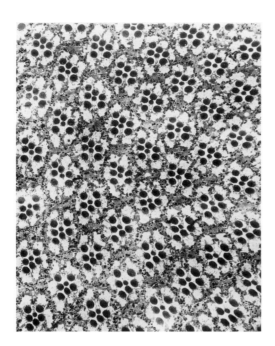

Plate 11 Retinal array of photoreceptors in fly. (Braitenberg and Kirschfeld, 1968.)

Plate 12 Dark field autoradiograph of part of the striate cortex in an adult macaque monkey in which the ipsilateral eye had been injected with tritiated proline-fucose 2 weeks previously. The areas labelled with radioactive atoms show up white. (Hubel and Wiesel, 1977.)

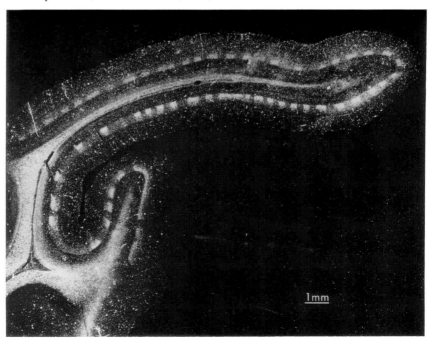

1mm

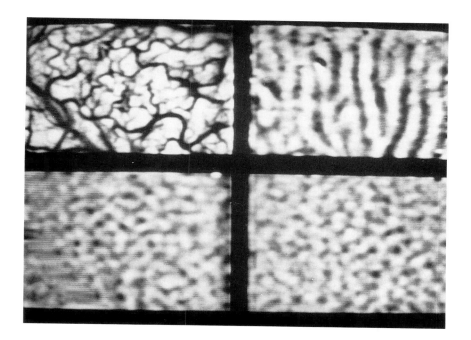

Plate 13 View from above of 8 mm patch of striate cortex, (a) as it appeared under white light, (b) showing ocular dominance bands produced by subtracting cortical images accumulated during visual stimulation of the contralateral eye from images accumulated during stimulation of the ipsilateral eye, (c) showing areas selectively sensitive to vertical orientations and (d) to oblique orientations of binocular stimuli. For images b, c and d illumination of the patch of cortex was at 720 nm since at this wavelength the blood vessels become virtually transparent. (Blasdel and Salama, 1986, reproduced by permission from *Nature* vol. 321, pp. 579–85. Copyright © 1986 Macmillan Magazines Ltd.)

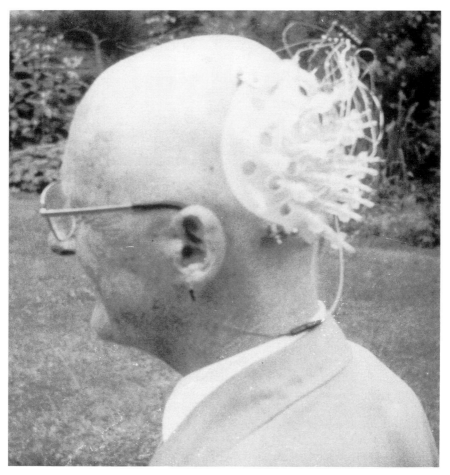

Plate 14 Author with array of 20 salt-pad electrodes mounted on a Perspex frame which is screwed to 3 feet glued to scalp. Figures 2.12 and 2.13 relate to this position of the electrodes. (MacKay, 1984a.)

Plate 15 Embossed Maltese crosses.

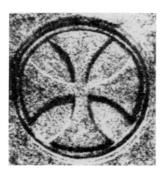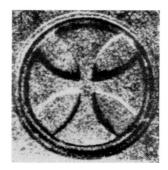

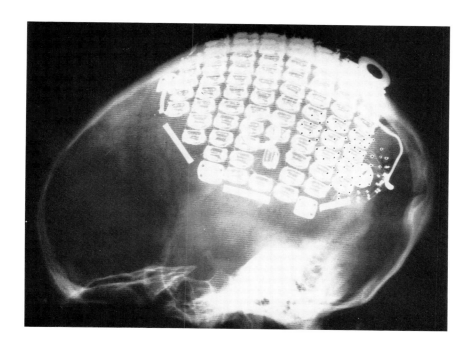

Plate 16 X-ray photographs of the head of patient with prototype visual prosthetic implant. Lateral and anterioposterior views. (Brindley and Lewin, 1968; Brindley, 1982, reproduced by permission of The Physiological Society.)

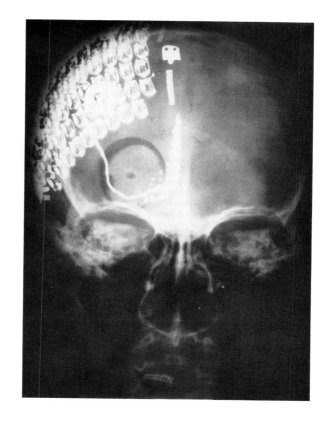

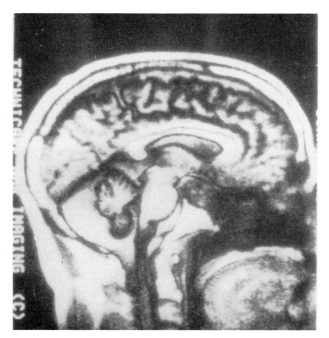

Plate 17 Nuclear magnetic resonance image of a sagittal section through the head. (Technicare NMR Imaging, 1983.)

Plate 18 A series of PET scans in a normal volunteer subject taken 2, 4, 6 and 8 cm above the orbital-meatal line depicting (top row) cerebral blood flow and (bottom row) uptake of oxygen. The middle row, being the ratio of the other two rows, represents the fractional extraction of oxygen. The subject was lying at rest. (Frackowiak, 1988.)

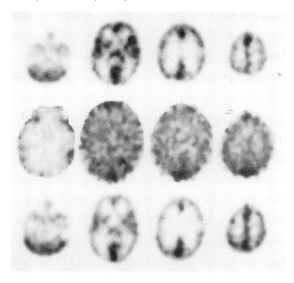

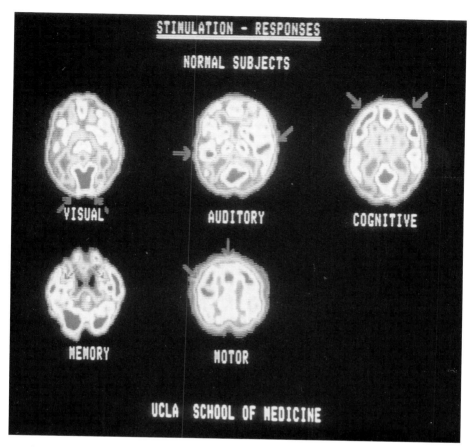

Plate 19 Near-horizontal PET scans at various levels through head during the performance of five tasks described in text. From left to right: visual, auditory, cognitive, memory and motor. (Phelps and Mazziotta, 1985; copyright 1985 by the American Association for the Advancement of Science.)

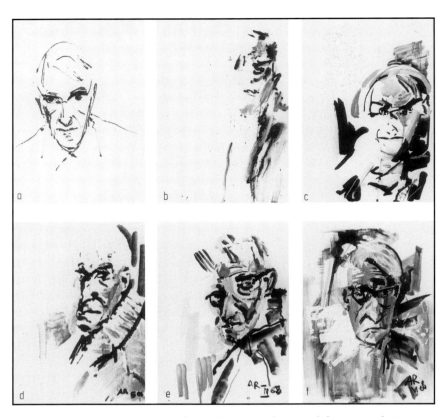

Plate 20 Left sided neglect after right parietal cortical lesion, and its compensation. Self-portraits by Anton Räderscheidt: (a) 2 years before, (b) 2 months, (c) $3\frac{1}{2}$, (d) 5, (e) 6, (f) 9 months after cerebral lesion. (Jung, 1974.)

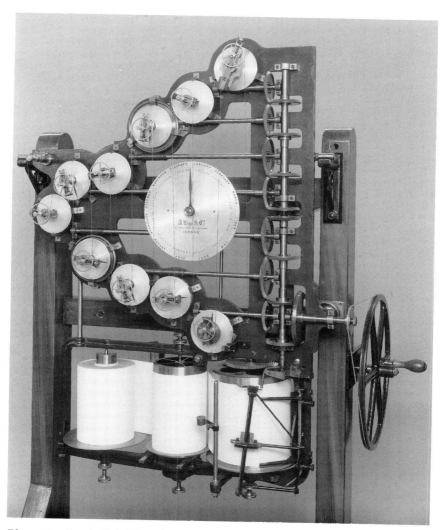

Plate 21 Lord Kelvin's tide predicter. (Thomson, 1881; reproduced by kind permission of the Trustees of the Science Museum, London.)

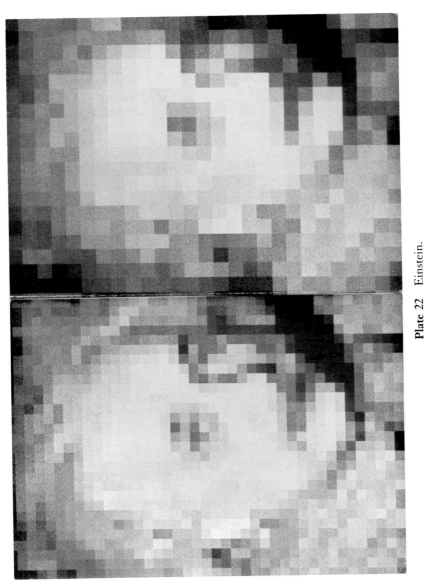

Plate 22 Einstein.

3

What are Brains for?

Looking at the structure of the brain, we have admired the immense complexity and detail of interconnection that it reveals under the microscope. Something like 10^{10} neurons each have on average perhaps 10^{14} contact points – which makes a hundred million million active connections within the structure of one human brain. In a quite reasonable sense, there is astronomical complexity inside every human head. But what we have been looking at is not just complexity. I mean, if you take a load of gravel and dump it on your drive you've got complexity. The striking thing about the brain is its *organized* complexity. That is the message we shall see again and again reinforced by the data we have picked up already. Brain science at the current level of detail and significance is only a few decades old; so we are only at its inception. But already it is abundantly clear that the brain, in the phrase from the Psalms which now is a kind of cliché, is 'fearfully and wonderfully made'. For many reasons the spectacle of our own brain is, of all the structures in the universe, a pre-eminent and proper object of wonder.

[*One of the most puzzling, indeed mysterious, things about the functioning of this intricate mass of protoplasm is the point noted and underlined in chapter 1: that the brain bears a special relation to what we think, experience and do. If we are to think about the question of what the brain is organized 'for', we must come back to this relationship – and to the conceptual gap – between the brain-story of unresting chemical and electrical activity, and the I-story of our own personal experience.*]

A conceptual gap

How relevant, you might ask, is the I-story to the brain-story or vice versa? One possible answer would be that the neurosciences as a whole are as irrelevant to cognitive science as knowledge about computer hardware is to the understanding of the program that the computer is following. If the computer is being used, let us say, to predict the weather or the economy, then understanding the inner workings of its semiconductors is of no help in grasping what is going on. There are people, in fact, who reject the idea that cognitive science needs any working relation with neuroscience on precisely those grounds.

I would argue that this is a mistake, based on a question-begging analogy [*the analogy of a digital computer*]: it is plausible only in relation to the kind of general-purpose symbol manipulator where, in principle, any physical configuration could be defined to have a given significance at the programming level, and neighbouring physical states can differ totally in symbolic significance. It is not true even of such a simple and familiar device as an analogue computer, where the physics of what is going on in the computer can be vitally relevant to the understanding of its mathematical function. The brain, I suspect, has an even closer relationship between its symbolic functioning and the physics and chemistry of what is going on inside it.

A second possible answer to our question, at the other extreme, would be that the neurophysiological explanation is the 'real thing', the only worthwhile explanation, which is destined one day to replace the old-fashioned 'pre-scientific' categories of conscious experience. When neurophysiology has fully matured, then, the analysis of cognition in subjective categories will wither away. Perhaps I don't need to argue that this view is also fallacious. It arises from a confusion of categories which in fact is quite well illustrated by the case of the computer itself. No-one in his senses would pretend that once we knew the physical explanation of the workings of a computer engaged in weather forecasting, speech recognition, chess or mathematics, we would have no further need for the categories of the programmer.

A conceptual bridge

What other possibilities are left? The suggestion I am going to explore is that we can best see the relevance of each story to the other if we adopt what I am going to call the information engineering approach. I mean the approach typical of the sort of scientist or engineer whose task is to devise or analyse ways of determining patterns of behaviour. What this does is to provide an intermediate conceptual level which offers in a certain sense a working link between the categories of conscious cognitive agency (to which the I-story refers) and those of neural activity (to which the brain-story refers).

As to how the gap is to be bridged, this is a challenge, not just to philosophy but to brain science itself, because, when you think about it, the brain as an object of scientific study is unique among all the other structures that science can look at in offering us two different kinds of clue to its workings. On the one hand there are all the physical and chemical and other clues that we have been talking about. But in addition there is the fact that the individual whose brain it is (if we are talking about the human brain) has conscious experience that he can talk about, bear witness to, and that we can study by the methods of experimental psychology. In some sense, that as yet we only dimly understand, this also must be a source of evidence as to what is going on in the depths of his brain. The temptation is to imagine that brain science ought to be particularly easy because we have this additional know-how: we know what it is like to be the possessor of a brain whose activity is, we suppose, responsible for our conscious experience. The question is: how can we make the link?

One point that I shall come back to many times is that it is very easy to make the links in the wrong way and quite difficult to produce, as it were, a fertile union between the studies of conscious experience on the one hand and the brain as a physico-chemical structure on the other.

Suggestions from automatic systems

Perhaps I may be autobiographical for a moment. I spent three years of the Second World War working on radar, and found myself drawn into brain research afterwards partly because during the war I had worked on the theory of automata and electronic computing and on the theory of information, all of which are highly relevant to such things as automatic pilots and automatic gun-direction. These are tasks which had formerly required human operators. Were there any limits, we used to ask ourselves, to the artificial simulation and eventual replacement of human beings in roles hitherto regarded as cognitive and intelligent?

I found myself grappling with problems in the design of artificial sense organs for naval gun-directors and with the principles on which electronic circuits could be used to simulate situations in the external world so as to provide goal-directed guidance for ships, aircraft, missiles and the like. [*As the radar dish rotates one wants to store and build up an unfading, increasingly reliable representation of the stationary and moving objects – rocks, ships and planes – which lie in each direction: some to be steered around, some to be aimed at.*]

The job of our radar systems was thus to supply information for the planning of action. What precisely did it mean to call something a 'representation'[1] of something else? Could this concept of 'information' be defined in sufficiently precise terms for scientific purposes? Could the overall process of the planning and execution of action be analysed in sufficiently abstract terms to allow each component to be conceived in mechanistic terms? If so, might this analysis then offer a theoretical framework for the understanding of the human cognitive process itself?

Later in the 1940s, when I was doing my PhD work, there was much talk of the brain as a computer and of the early digital computers that were just making the headlines as 'electronic brains'. As an analogue computer man I felt pretty strongly convinced that the brain, whatever it was, was not a digital computer. I didn't think it was an analogue computer either in the conventional sense. But this naturally rubbed under my skin the question: well, if it is not either of these, what kind of a system is it? Is there any way of following through the kind of analysis that is appropriate to these artificial automata so as to understand better the kind of system that the human brain is? That was the beginning of my slippery slope into brain research.

The brain: an information system

Of course there is one short answer, which is inevitably partial, but which has turned out to be a very fruitful one for many of us. The brain, whatever else it is, is a system which in addition to running on energy, as every biological system has to do, runs in an important and practical sense on *information*. Because the technology of radar and the like had led us to make quite precise what we mean by saying that a system runs on information (needs a certain amount of information to do a particular job and so on), we felt encouraged to hope that following through that level of analysis of brain function could be profitable.

[*For the next few pages we take an excursion into information-flow systems and the reader may wonder whether we have lost sight of both the brain and first-hand experience! What we are looking for is a bridge that can span the conceptual gap and link brain and experience. The language and ideas of information theory have the right kind of hybrid status to provide a vocabulary of (rigorous) concepts which latch on to the physiological concepts of the brain-story on the one hand and also to the characteristic concerns of the I-story on the other. At the level of physiology it is clearly not inappropriate to talk in engineering terms – the circuits in living systems exist to do various jobs. But what about the I-story?*

Here it may be helpful to bear in mind that one of our most characteristic conscious activities is the pursuit of goals, the sizing up of likely outcomes and the revision of goals. As is said later: 'If we ask what ... distinguishes us most from sticks and stones and other objects ... the answer is ... our capacity to evaluate – to attach the label good and bad, to say "I like this, I don't want that". We assess events or situations, both real and hypothetical, as desirable/undesirable, good/bad, plus/minus.' Conscious agents evaluate.

Moreover to achieve our goals, however abstract, we generally have to do something. We reach out our hand and arm in order to grasp something we fancy, we turn our heads and eyes so as to bring within our visual grasp something that has caught our attention, we make the highly skilled muscular performances of speech. Even when we take no immediate action, we are set up ready for action should need arise. This emphasis on preparedness *for activity in the world as the object of our internal activities leads us, as we shall see, to think of our faculties as being a seamless whole with our activities. Our senses, our memory, our abstractive abilities, are not best understood in isolation: they are bound up with our readiness for bodily activity in the world. In what follows, the topics of perception, learning, concept formation and originality, even when not explicitly mentioned, are never far away. They have been very much in mind in the hammering out over the years of the integrated understanding sketched below.*

In building his bridge between brain and experience Donald MacKay is constantly aware of the material in which the foundations at both ends must be embedded. On the physiological side there are those massive random-looking cross-connections, the multitude of feedback connections, those 'shivers' of subtly changing voltage fed down the dendrites, the continuously variable factors that are present in the conductivities of axons and synapses, besides the concentrations of all the surrounding chemicals. Looking towards the I-story side, he sets himself the task of finding enough room for (among other things) the obvious facts of remembering and development, of tacit knowledge and of originality. He is seeking too a functional distinction between conscious and unconscious activity, between reception and perception and between the various meanings, intended and received, of a message.]

Control: action under evaluation

To give you a feeling for what one means by a system that runs on information let us consider figure 3.1, which brings out a number of points which I wish to make. It shows the bare bones of a thermostat, or indeed of a whole range of possible automatic mechanisms for pursuing a particular goal actively by correcting, automatically, conditions that lead away from the goal and helping trends towards the goal.

Its basic components are three:

1   There is an *effector system*, E, something for producing effects in the field of action, F: this would be a heater and/or cooler in the case of a thermostat. The 'keyboard' is a way of showing diagrammatically that the effector has a repertoire of possible modes of action – to heat or to cool.

2   Then, in order that the system should take note of what is going on in its field of action, it needs a *receptor system*, R, which provides an indication I_f of the state of the field, under as many categories as necessary (for the thermostat, that of temperature). R will therefore indicate, among other things, the effects that E is having on the state

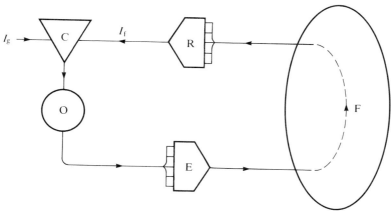

Figure 3.1 Simple negative feedback loop, as exemplified in self-governing systems such as an oven thermostat, Watt's steam governor, automatic pilot, etc. The action of the effector system, E, in the field, F, is monitored by the receptor system, R, which provides an indication I_f of the state of F. This indication is compared with the goal criterion I_g in the comparator, C, which informs the organizing system, O, of any mismatch. O selects from the repertoire of E action calculated to reduce the mismatch.

of F. In the case of a thermostat R would be perhaps a simple mechanical thermometer, a piece of bimetal strip, which moves a lever one way if the temperature goes up and the other way if the temperature goes down.

So far we have got two devices which we would have in any house without anything automatic going on. You could turn the heater/cooler up or down, on or off, by hand and you could read the thermometer yourself.

3 *Evaluation*. What the thermostat does, as we all know, is to take the indication of the state of the field, and feed it into a very simple little box which we usually call the evaluator or comparator, C, because it compares the indicated temperature against a 'goal' temperature set by the householder. This estimates the degree of 'mismatch' (or match) between the actual state of the field F (I have called the indication of this state I_f) and its goal or target state, as set by I_g. On the basis of that difference it produces what the engineer would usually call a 'mismatch' signal. (That's a bit pessimistic because it may be a match signal!) The mismatch signal can be either

positive or negative (and may indicate also the extent of the mismatch).

From this match/mismatch information it should be possible to determine the form of action by the effector E (for example, heating or cooling) required to correct for any indicated departure of F from its target state. The job of calculating the corrective action we assign to an 'organizing system', O, whose output then supplies the information needed by E. In a simple thermostat O need be no more than a lever linking the movements of a mechanical thermometer to a switch that turns on the heater, or the cooler. We must ensure, of course, that the lever works the right way – heating when the temperature is too low and vice versa – otherwise feedback will be positive and the system will run amok!

Steam engines had the first of these man-made automatic governors to be widespread. It was James Watt's governor that was treated by Clerk-Maxwell as the first mathematical problem in what is now called the theory of automation. The point, first understood in those days of steam engines, was that you didn't have to have a small boy whose job was to work the control at E so as to bring that mismatch between I_f and I_g to zero: you could take the indication of mismatch itself and tie it appropriately to the selector from the repertoire of action and by doing that you would be able to organize automatically the corrections that are needed.

I say 'automatically', but in something more complicated than a thermostat an appropriate selection by O from the repertoire of action may be highly complicated. An automatic pilot, for example, has to keep an aircraft on a level keel in spite of the bumps of turbulence, cross-winds and so on. In such a device there will be several degrees of freedom, several dimensions, in which controls can be altered. I_f is thus distributed over many sensory channels. Match/mismatch may have to be estimated under several simultaneous criteria, and the repertoire of action involved may be so elaborate that powerful calculations have to be continuously performed in O if landing is to be successful. Furthermore, in situations where alternative sequences or strategies become more appropriate as circumstances change, a major problem for the designers of such systems is how to provide the information that will select the appropriate option.

Nevertheless the basic principle is the same in all these self-regulating loops: the indication of mismatch is used to instigate and to select organizing activity calculated to bring about a change in the world, the field of action, which will then reduce the mismatch between the indicated state and the goal state.

Agency

The basic feedback loop of figure 3.1 represents a very simple mechanism that certainly has no claim to be conscious, or anything like that. But we notice two things about it: it is a system that runs on information and it is also a goal-directed agent. What I want to underline is that talking about agency – which is *activity under evaluation*, activity in view of an end or purpose or goal – does not presuppose consciousness. You can have artificial agency in a system which to the best of our knowledge is not at all a conscious being in the sense that you and I are. There is no tendency for the designers of thermostats to think of them as people with an I-story to tell! But they do have agency and they do have power actively to resist changes in the world, including changes brought about by people, which disturb their pursuit of the goal.

If you open the oven door, the gas flame immediately comes up to fight you and to try to keep the temperature back at the level specified by the dial setting. If somebody moves around in a light aircraft so that the plane left to itself would tilt, then the automatic pilot automatically resists what is being done. There are lots of situations in which things may go wrong and you find yourself actively struggling with an automatic agent of this sort as if it were a living, conscious being. You can have nowadays sophisticated agents whose field of action is a chess board. Exactly the same basic flow map describes how this system can move pieces around on the chess board in such a way as to have the goal of defeating an adversary at chess – with no pretence, I insist, that there is anybody there, conscious of you as you are conscious of what is going on on the board. There is simply the succession of automatic chains of feedback based on flow of information.

Insights at the information level: causation and explanation

Let us spell out a bit more what we mean by 'flow of information' because this is quite crucial for later discussions. When we say, for example, that there is a flow of information from the receptor (e.g. the thermometer) to the comparator, what we mean is that the *form* of the input to the comparator is determined by the *form* of the change of temperature at the receptor, regardless of where the energy comes from.

Take a simpler example: somebody comes to the front door and presses the button in his own characteristic rhythm, 'ta-ta-ta-tum-tum'. That has a particular form. The bell in the kitchen obediently replicates that form. The person at the door has determined the form of the bell's activity in the kitchen; but he has not supplied the energy. The energy comes from a transformer in the kitchen.

Form determining form gives rise to *information flow*, or if you like, exemplifies information flow. Force determining force (which is what physics is about) can involve a flow of energy in the opposite direction. Information goes from the front door to the kitchen; energy flows from the kitchen out to the front door button and back again. Flow of energy and flow of information are two quite different notions: they can have opposite directions and they can have very little to do with each other, except that you must (generally) have some flow of energy if you are going to have a flow of information. [*There* can *be cases when information flows although no energy flows: the non-arrival of a hoped-for letter, or a silent telephone, may convey a great deal of information.*]

Explanation at more than one level

You can trace chains of cause and effect at either level. What information technology has brought into being as a self-conscious discipline in this century is a new level of causal analysis additional to the classical level of physics. In classical physics, as we all know, the basic concept is energy: the flow of energy is what you look to in order to explain events. In the level of information and control-analysis you have – in addition to whatever flow of energy is going on – a flow of information. You can have causal explanations, chains of cause and effect, at the informational level. You can ask, for example: why is this unhappy aircraft tilting, rocking like a see-saw, all the time? The answer is: because some delay has got into its feedback loop. It is a very common disease of a self-regulating system: if the feedback loop gets sticky, so that a correction takes too long to take effect, then things have got worse before the correction comes, and swung too far the other way. Another example would be the cycle of booms and slumps in the classical market disease. This oscillation is explained by saying that the information flow path has too long a delay. The cure for it (in the simple situation) is to shorten the delay. As you shorten the delay the oscillations get faster and smaller and finally the thing settles. You then say: I have now *understood* what is going on and I have understood it in terms of information flow.

Notice there is not the slightest hint of rivalry between that (information engineering) explanation and the explanation that a physicist would give of what every element in the loop is doing. When the engineer says 'it was the delay that caused the trouble', he is not saying 'you physicists would talk about electric currents and forces, but of course I have got the real thing, and you were talking nonsense', or 'I have a rival explanation and I hope mine will win and yours will wither'. He knows that the physical explanation must be there if his story is true. This is what I would mean by saying that causal analysis at the level of information flow is complementary to and not a rival of the kind of causal analysis at the physical level that classical physics has accustomed us to.

The new discipline of information science and the information technology that goes with it thus introduce us to the idea of multiple levels of determination, and they do so in a very hard-nosed way. People's money has to be made, their reputations gained or lost, on the correctness of explanations and diagnoses made at the information-flow level, which are not in the least rendered either out of date or rivals by the fact that there exist physical explanations for all that every individual entity in the loop is doing. You need *both* because you would miss the point being made in the information-flow analysis if you didn't carry it through in addition to the stories that the physicist correctly tells about the physical causes and effects in each of the elements of the system.

This is a major point which we shall keep coming back to: that in thinking about systems that handle information we are thinking about a situation which has more than one level of causation without any rivalry between the levels. They are situations in which determination ('A determines B') can be instantiated at more than one level without any suggestion that the one determinative explanation is the 'real' one and the others are 'nothing but' something else.

Agency – unconscious and conscious

This brings us to the question: how far can flow systems of this sort be pressed into service to cover the full range of human and animal activity? So far I have stressed that these devices, when we build them, have no claim to be conscious. But not only do you and I know for a fact that we individually are conscious: I think that we would be perverse and counter-intuitive if we denied that many higher animals are conscious too. So conscious agency (which includes goal-directed agency as a typical case) is widespread, and the question that we are bound to ask ourselves is: if we try to use this kind of information-flow analysis, is there any kind of pointer as to what has got to come in, in order to make the necessary distinction between agency that is unconscious and agency that is conscious?

To bring it nearer home, the human body contains not just one, but a whole hierarchy of regulative mechanisms, many of them with flow loops like that in figure 3.1. The pupil of your eye is an example. I don't know if you have ever played the following game but it is quite fun. Take a piece of smooth card, poke two pinholes in it about 1/8th inch apart and hold them close in front of one eye. Two bright circles, images of the pupil, will be seen. If you now vary the amount of light entering the other eye by opening and closing it, you will find that the images of the pinholes change in size. Each time the other eye is illuminated the circles shrink. The pupils of the two eyes work in joint harness and automatically adjust to the intensity of the light reaching them.

The interesting thing is that you are totally unconscious that this pupil adjustment is going on. This is *unconscious agency* within part of your own body. There is a real distinction then between those goal-directed actions under evaluation that occur in our own bodies but do not, as we might say, generate conscious experience and those that do. So within the human body we need a distinction – an operational distinction – between conscious agency and unconscious agency, between the kind of explanation that would make sense of conscious agency and that which would explain unconscious agency.

Action on the springs of action: supervisory activity

Now what I want to show in figure 3.2 is the first minimal addition that it seems to me would be necessary if our flow system were to be elaborated so as to begin to take cognizance of this distinction. So far our system has been a slave. It depends on an outside source for the specification of its goal, I_g. Before we can begin to approximate to autonomous cognitive agency we must introduce a system at a higher level, whose function is to determine and order the priorities of the goals to be pursued. I have called it the supervisory system, SS. [*In the case of our thermostat we are thinking of the supervisory function exercised by the housewife when she decides, let us say, to abandon her previous policy of economy and to set the goal-temperature in view of her household's state of health, rather than solely with her eye on the fuel bill.*]

A characteristic thing about all the systems we have been discussing – automatic pilot, thermostats and the like – is that they have something ending in free space. The thermostat has a knob waiting for the housewife to come and set it; the automatic pilot has a knob waiting for the pilot to come and set it; but a living organism is not normally so equipped. There is a great deal of its activity in which the system must set its own goals. As human brains don't have knobs for other people to set, the setting of goals must be a function of some of the structures within the same system – if the system is a self-consistent information-flow system. You realize I am not being dogmatic here: we have no idea how far the human brain obeys physical laws even – but we are working on the assumption that it does and that for its informational activities it requires information. So if we ask where the information comes *from* to determine a change in goal setting, the answer is: it comes from another part of the system. So we draw a box which we label supervisory system, simply to indicate that fact of life, as it were, from the standpoint of information engineering. It's not that we know where to look in the brain for a box with this function, but it is something which is a necessity of the flow map.

Notice that in adding these minimal flow lines in figure 3.2 we are not so much building a theory as representing facts we already know. We are not saying: I wonder if it is like this? We are doing something which comes from the other end. We know for a fact that people do certain things. For example, they are struggling to achieve a certain target and the question occurs to them: should we give up and change our goal? Or an animal has the goal of drinking water at a water-hole and out of the corner of its eye sees a predator approaching. The question must arise for it, although not in so many words: shall I continue to pursue the goal of ingesting water or shall I switch goals so as to take to flight? This kind of goal-switching process, and the computations behind it, count as supervisory activity.

These are facts, as far as we know; certainly they are facts about ourselves. If we draw information-flow maps which represent no more than these facts we are not generating a theory; we are trying to be obedient to our data in a certain language. You see the difference? A theory is something for which you would not get evidence unless you made a test to see whether the theory fits. But when you use this kind of flow map you are using a graphical language to try to do justice to facts (like 'fight or flight') that you have already got. This doesn't mean that you are excused from making tests, but the tests have a different kind of function. They are really tests of how accurately you have represented what you already know; so there is a slight difference in the logic.

The supervisory system and its links

The supervisory system, SS, has, in short, the power to change the target settings I_g so as to settle for a new target because of some unacceptable mismatch being signalled to it from the comparator C.

A second area where action by SS could be valuable is that of the organizing system O. O's job, we remember, is to determine as quickly and accurately as possible the action required by E to bring I_f into line with the target I_g. It is a computational network in some general sense such that in response to a mismatch signal it selects from the repertoire an action calculated to have a good chance of bringing the indicated state into line with the goal state. The subroutines within the repertoire (in a sense that we shall speak more about below and in later chapters) represent implicitly the constraints of reality, the structure of the field of action, F, against which the system is struggling.

In order that this representation should be kept up to date, the organizing system needs sensory information. So I have drawn the

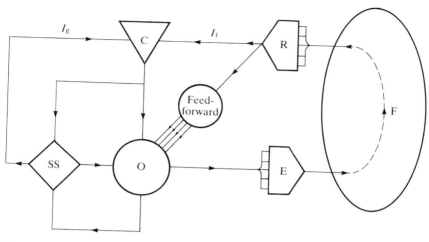

Figure 3.2 Information-flow map of a system capable of modifying its own goals. SS, supervisory system; C, comparator; O, organizing system; F, field of action; E, effectors; R, receptors; FF, feedforward; I_f, indicated state of field; I_g, indicated goal-state or criterion of evaluation. The organizing system, O, organizes the repertoire of possible activity (e.g. fight, feeding or flight) which may be pre-wired and/or built up in response to the regularities of its field of action, F. The supervisory system, SS, selects from O part of the repertoire appropriate to incoming mismatch signals from the comparator, C, and supervises the development and trial and updating of the repertoire. [(*Readers who wonder why this particular flow map is preferred to alternative candidates are referred to MacKay (1962, 1965a) and to p. 79. It is a matter of informational economy – the avoidance of duplication.*)]

route labelled feedforward, FF, where one line on the diagram is probably millions of channels from the receptors. The clues from the receptors are processed in advance and as a guide to the action actually taken.

In most cases of course the information from the receptors about some feature of the world will not be in a form that determines straightforwardly the 'formula' to be used by O in planning relevant action with respect to it. The sophisticated operation of revising the organizing structure in matching response to the receptor information coming in requires organizing activity at a higher level. This, then, is the second respect in which we can see the supervisory system as being needed.

The task for the supervisory system is thus to derive and impose constraints on the operation of O to match the demands extracted by the sensory feedforward system FF, this keeping the organizing system O up to date in its readiness to take account of the structure of its world. The constraints will in general amount to hypotheses as to the state of readiness that will best match the external situation indicated by the sensory feedforward, and SS will have to be flexible in response to indications that its current hypothesis needs to be revised.

So we have in figure 3.2 a hierarchic organization: while the organizing system O has as its field of action the external world F, the supervisory system treats the internal organizing network O as its field of action, receiving feedback from it and supplying feedforward as well as acting directly on its goal settings.

For our purpose in this book the full technicalities are not important. What matters is that we are finding here a way of systematically mapping the lines of cause and effect that link the flow of information in a system which now has some of the capacities of the human being to select his own goals, to change his goals and goal priorities in the light of experience of what it is like to pursue the current goal. It becomes, in other words, a system which becomes its own master. In the sense in which the housewife is the master (or mistress) of the thermostat, this system is its own master or mistress.

The organizing system: profiting from redundancy

[*Since the organizing system is not the primary concern of the present chapter the paragraph which follows may be skipped and returned to later. It is included here to fill out figure 3.2 for those who wish to gain a clearer picture of this lower level, whose goals and repertoire of alternative activities the supervisory level is to supervise.*]

If the field F had no stable structure, the system could only feel its way towards its goal by successive approximations, and would be quite at a loss in a rapidly changing field. If, however, the demands imposed by the field exhibit any stable or regular features, such as those arising from the alternation of day and night, then of course the selective operation on the effectors, E, could in principle be partly prefabricated; we could imagine incorporating, for example, a time switch in the organizer O to replicate those components of the selective operation that are predictable on the basis of the regularity. The organizer may in part act upon feedforward from the receptive system (for example, a second thermometer outside the building, registering ambient temperature), or it may simply abstract from the output of the comparator those regular features that become predictable. In either case this organizer, which prefabricates as much of the selective operation as matches the regularity of the demand, in a sense *represents* internally the regular feature of the outside world against which it is struggling. If, for example, an immovable object lies in front of a robot, the repertoire in O should be so organized as to exclude actions leading to collisions and to include subroutines for circumnavigating it.

Consciousness requires self-supervisory activity

In all this we are not of course talking about boxes but *systems*. The supervisory system covers the whole group of information-processing elements so linked as to exercise control of planning, representation and evaluation, including evaluation of its own criteria of evaluation. During conscious control of external action this system will extend out through the organizing system into the external world: in its functioning entirety it may not be confined within the boundaries of the agent's skin. A blind man probing with his cane, for example, feels the world out there at the tip of his cane. There is a clear sense in which *he* could claim to be consciously in contact with the object he is probing. If we want to identify the informational system whose activity is the correlate of his conscious activity, we must be prepared to find it extending right through to the tip of his cane. What is implied by lettering a box 'supervisory system', however, is that if that particular structure were knocked out of action, then supervisory activity would be impossible. No matter how elaborate the degree of sensory–motor coordination shown by the remainder of the nervous system (remember the pupillary reflex), there would be no *running review of current priorities* in the manner that is characteristic of conscious agency. The priority-determining process would be 'frozen'.

Here, in this supervisory activity, it seems to me that we have an information-flow structure with some of the necessary features to serve as a direct correlate of our conscious experience. The most characteristic aspect of being conscious, as we all know at first hand, is that we both evaluate the ongoing state of affairs and determine or revise at will our goal priorities and criteria of evaluation. To 'give one's mind to' some current activity means primarily to evaluate it and its foreseen implications. To fail to do so does not necessarily mean that we fail to react to stimuli, but rather that we fail to evaluate their implications.

I have said all this not with a view to concluding that such a re-entrant information-flow structure is a sufficient condition for conscious experience, but in order to suggest that this kind of supervisory hierarchy is a *necessary* condition, in hard-nosed engineering terms, for any conscious experiencing that does occur. As we shall see later, there are quite a number of contexts of brain research where this kind of distinction has practical consequences. If I am right, then the search for an 'anatomical substrate of consciousness' is not meaningless; but the direct correlate of a specific experience would not be the activity of specific neurons, but rather the presence of a correspondingly specific information-flow pattern. Note, moreover, that this pattern of supervisory agency is a *systemic* entity, which is associable only with the supervisory structure as a whole – in the sense in which the 'howl' that develops when a microphone is too near its loudspeaker is a systemic entity, associable only with the resulting positive feedback loop as a whole: the howl does not have its origin in any one of the chain of components, but in the loop set up by allowing the amplifier to supply its own input. Similarly, I suggest, conscious experience does not have its origin in any one of the participating brain nuclei, but in the positive feedback chain-mesh that is set up when the evaluative system *becomes its own evaluator.*

[*The previous few paragraphs have been concerned with the assessment and switching of goals, with an eye all the time on the human cognitive agent. But some readers may have been restively wanting to ask whether a mechanical system really could embody something as abstract as the faculty of judgement? The following section has been inserted (from MacKay, 1967) to show the lines on which hardware can be envisaged for weighing rival goals against each other in the light of 'higher' goals.*]

Judgement – and good judgement?

Obviously the supervisory system embodies norms. Our thermostat, for example, might be provided with a supervisory system that could be said to have 'economy' as its overriding norm: its setting of I_g might be tied mechanically to a meter which reads the average rate of fuel consumption, and a clock which is set to take advantage of off-peak tariffs. It would then pursue as a goal the maintenance of a temperature 'within its means', actively opposing large short term fluctuations from the goal temperature, but 'lowering its sights' if the long term demand on its resources proved too great.

Given a normative criterion or goal we can thus specify fairly readily an information-flow system to organize appropriate behaviour. We know what we mean by a 'good' or 'efficient' method of organizing the pursuit of ends. What, however, we do not understand, in anything like the same sense, is the process by which our criteria themselves are formed and adjusted. Suppose, for example, that a further factor were evaluated, such as the stability of the target temperature. We can envisage an indicator of the variation of the goal-setting (say its root mean square, or r.m.s.). Here we have a potential conflict of norms, since in a changing environment demand on resources will be high if the goal is not adjusted from time to time, whereas the r.m.s. variation will be high if it is readjusted. How is the system to inter-relate these two? Can we meaningfully ask: how *ought* the system to relate them?

Various possibilities spring to mind. We could arrange for a simple 'tug of war' or mechanical balance between the two evaluative signals of 'economy' and 'stability', so that the system would always find a compromise 'goal-policy'. The relative weights given to each would be determined by the strengths of coupling of the two signals to the balancing mechanism (figure 3.3). Alternatively the combination of the two might be non-linear, so that, for example, the criterion of stability had priority over economy at low levels of fuel consumption, but at high levels economy became overriding.

The point I want to make is two-fold. First, there is no difficulty in finding a mechanical analogue of processes of the nature of judgement; but secondly, nothing in our specification of the case, as far as I can see, can enable us to evaluate one process as better or more rational *in itself* than another. As Sir Geoffrey Vickers has put it: 'Men, institutions and societies learn what to want as well as how to get, what to be as well as what to do and the two forms of adaptation are closely connected.... The norms which men pursue and the problems which they try to solve are largely self-set by a partly conscious process which merits ... more study than it has yet received.... It can con-

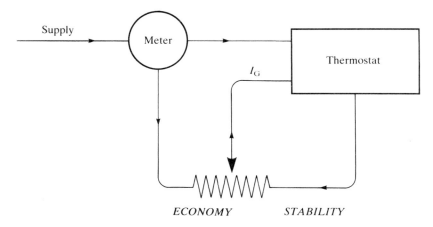

Figure 3.3 A simple system embodying a judgement about the relative importance of the goals of economy and stability.

veniently be studied in the overt processes of public life where it is more than usually explicit.'

The decision to adopt one form of coupling (of the norms) is a decision to *be* one kind of organism in preference to another. Only if we accept an external criterion of what makes a *good organism* can we begin to evaluate it. It may be agreed, for example, that a system (returning to our heater) that undervalues economy will not last long, so that natural selection may in any case bring about the predominance of one evaluative policy rather than another. But is longevity then to be accepted as unquestionably the ultimate good? Merely to raise the question is to demonstrate the bankruptcy of logical deduction as a substitute for ultimate evaluation (MacKay, 1967).

Of course, there must somewhere be criteria which are not open to revision. In the case of living organisms these criteria include such things as the level of carbon dioxide in the blood – which if departed from sufficiently would lead to convulsions or other breakdowns. So in drawing the system which sets its own goals we are not suggesting that this is a system which could pursue any goal whatsoever. Its range of goal pursuits and adjustments of targets and criteria are limited physiologically all along the line and it is only within certain ranges that the system can be in that sense self-supervisory and self-targeting.

Mind and brain

I realize that in assuming, all this while, that the brain is a completely autonomous system, I may seem to have been ignoring the position strongly advocated by such distinguished thinkers as Sir Karl Popper and Sir John Eccles, whose famous book *The Self and its Brain* (1977) suggests in effect that the human brain must have some special point at which it is open to the non-physical or quasi-physical influence of the 'mind'. 'The self', says Popper, 'in a sense plays on the brain, as a pianist plays on a piano or a driver plays on the controls of a car.' In terms of our flow map, I think it would be just at the input I_g to the evaluator that they would expect to find mental influences coming in from another 'world'.

I agree of course that in ordinary speech we would say that the setting of my goal criteria is one of the functions of my 'mind'. If I 'change-my-mind', then my current goals and norms change accordingly. So let us return to the question with which this chapter began. How are we to think of the facts of the I-story and brain-story as related? What kind of relationship are we homing in on between the events and facts to which the I-story bears witness (those private but indubitable events and conditions that we call 'seeing', 'hearing', 'believing', 'liking' and 'changing our minds') and the kind of events to which the brain story bears witness? Given that the I-story points to data which are happenings that we would be lying to deny, given that the brain-story points to data which we would be at least mistaken to deny – how are we to think of those happenings as related? This question takes us into the heart of a topic of closest relevance to the concern of the Gifford lecture series and there is, as I am sure you know, a whole spectrum of tentative answers.

Interactionist dualism

One extreme I have mentioned above; it would describe itself as 'interactionist dualism'. Dualism here means believing that there are at least two worlds of reality: one world is the physical world; another, the typical dualist would say, is the 'world of the mind'. The interactionist dualist would picture the mind as a non-physical occupant, in some almost literal sense, of the mental world (a world other than the physical world), and would postulate interaction between the two.

This view is associated classically with the name of Descartes but it has modern exponents in varied forms. I mentioned above Sir John Eccles, a Nobel prize winner in neurophysiology. In 1986 he produced a paper which puts very clearly one way of trying to answer our question: how are these related? It is entitled 'Do mental events cause neural events analogously to the probability fields of quantum mechanics?' The basic question is: do mental events *cause* neural events, in the kind of way that one physical situation can cause another physical situation? Should we, in other words, answer our question by saying that these two worlds interact causally through some unknown quasi-physical interference by one world on the other? His hypothesis is that 'a non-material mental event, such as an intention to move, could influence the subtle probabilistic operations of synaptic boutons'. Synaptic boutons are at the contact points onto those spines that we looked at (in figures 2.2 and 2.5 and plates 6–9) which link cells to one another and, as I stressed, these are very important determinants of the behaviour of the whole system. There are 10^{14} of them determining by and large how the whole system dances. So Eccles's hypothesis is that the mind, in a non-physical world, influences the fine scale, the electron scale, mechanics by which the chemicals are spat across the synapses onto the region of the receiving cells.

This interactionist view does have a number of advocates today, and is not in that sense out of date, although I think it is fair to say, and Eccles would agree, that he is in a relatively small minority in espousing this model. Here I would suggest that, although we may be able to fit in all the facts of experience, we buy into a whole array of unresolved questions, for example: (a) how can it be that an immaterial 'world of the mind' can interact with the brain; and (b) what evidence at all is there that the brain is subject to influences other than those operating in any given locality from the physical environment and the forces it exerts?[2] In other words, I would argue that I see no need to go to the ontological extreme of postulating 'two worlds' with some kind of unexplained interaction between them.

Epiphenomenalism and other varieties of materialism

At the other extreme of the spectrum of views there is the sort of view that is usually called epiphenomenalism. What this view asserts is the ineffectiveness of the mind or mental events in relation to the physical brain activity. I think it was T. H. Huxley who said that the activity of the mind bears as little efficacious relation to the workings of the brain as the sound of the whistle of a steam locomotive bears to the workings of the engine. The 'mind', if you want to insist that there is such a thing, is a kind of dangler that makes noises, but the system is just going along with no interference, certainly, and indeed no significant dependence on what the mind is up to.

[*A neighbouring view from that end of the spectrum would be: 'I am not happy with the line down the middle of table 1.1 because these terms "I see, I hear", etc. are simply our way of expressing in words particular states of neural activity in the second column'.*]

Along this spectrum, and it may be a spectrum with more than one dimension, there are many variations. Many people, for example, would want to label their position 'materialist'. Some people call themselves emergentist materialists, others reductionist materialists, but the main emphasis would be on the primacy of the material. They would say that what is essentially going on is matter in motion. They might say that mental properties 'emerge' from this in the way that the properties of a molecule emerge from the atoms that you bring together in a compound – but in the end the reality is matter.

The primacy of the I-story

'In the end the reality is matter.' I think I ought to comment on this at this stage: it is something we shall be coming back to frequently. The idea that you have to set these things in a pecking order seems to me to be at the very least premature and sometimes quite perverse. But if there were any suggestion of a pecking order between the data of the I-story and the data of the brain-story, then as a matter of simple fact it is the I-story that comes first. Materialism as a posture has reality standing on its head, for what we know first and foremost are the facts of the I-story. Our conscious experience is the platform upon which even our doubting must be based, a point, by the way, first made not by Descartes, although he often gets the credit for it, but by Augustine of Hippo many centuries earlier. If I doubt even my own existence, by doubting I have established my own existence. But this is my own existence as a cognitive agent. We would not know anything about brains, we certainly would not have any basis for talking with confidence about brains, unless we had conscious experience to provide us with the evidence (through experienced sights and so on) that there *are* brains. So if there were any fight between these two for priority, I think it is perfectly clear that ontologically as well as epistemologically the I-story comes first.

To the materialist quoted above who expressed himself unhappy with the line between the two columns of table 1.1 on the grounds that the first column is 'simply our way of expressing things that are going on in our brain', I would say: 'O come, nonsense! You and I have absolutely no idea what is going on in our brains. Absolutely none. So to accuse me or yourself of expressing in other words things that are going on in our brains is nonsense. We know nothing about it. As conscious agents we *do* know that, for instance, I see someone in front of me listening to the sound of my voice. These experiences are something I would be lying to deny. So I do know them. But that there happens to be any correlation between those experiences and things going on in my head is an empirical matter which astonishes me and fascinates me and of which I still don't know any of the details. It would be quite wrong to say that I am only choosing other words to express these facts but perversely chose subjective terms to express them. "I see ... I hear ..." are data. They are not optional extras or alternatives to something else, they are things which I would be lying to deny. Among the things which I see, etc., are the facts about brains and in particular the facts about this brain. In that sense the whole of the brain story is nested within the I-story.'

Having said this, I think that it is a silly game to pit these two against one another. As I have been trying to suggest and shall be arguing further, they are harmoniously complementary. The one is spelling out the *personal* significance of a unitary situation, another aspect of which is dealt with in the brain-story.

To those who hear me as saying that the two columns offer two different descriptions of the 'same thing' at different levels I would offer the following point. If an equation has two roots, and it is embodied in a computer, then the facts about the equation are not facts about the computer – except in a Pickwickian sense. Computers don't have roots! And yet, if the computer is solving the equation there is a direct physical correlate for the statement 'the equation has two roots', and any engineer can tell you what it is. Certainly there is *correlation*, and there are isomorphisms in it, but it is not a translation.

The importance of our material embodiment

I would not want to suggest that our identity is as unrelated to the matter of our brains as, for example, the equation that a computer solves is unrelated to the matter that a computer is built of. We all know that you can have an IBM computer or a DEC computer built out of quite different stuff and they will solve the same equation in the same way. I am not at all suggesting that the particular embodiment doesn't matter: we shall see much evidence to the contrary. But I am going to be suggesting that when we speak of mental activity (as I would wish to do) as *efficacious* in determining, sometimes, the form of our action, we have no more reason to imagine that there is interference going on with the physics of our brains than we do in the case of an equation which determines the form of the behaviour of a computer.

If we program a computer to solve a certain equation, we all know what it means to say that its behaviour is *determined*, for the time being, by that equation and no other. But this does not in the least mean that when you analyse the physics of a computer you expect to find elements sensitive to 'influences' from a 'mathematical world' which are somehow interfering with the functioning.

In summary, I shall be insisting that matter matters: that the matter of our brains, as well as the informational program embodied in our brains, is important to what and who we are. Nevertheless, looking at what we know about ourselves, it is quite clear that we are first and foremost persons with an I-story to tell and it is as part of that body of facts that we have a well-founded belief that we are also physical objects that have a claim to be reckoned with as objects in the physical world.

Comprehensive realism

What I'm going to be suggesting might be called a recognition of duality without the extreme of dualism. I think it is undeniable that conceptually there is a duality here. The concepts of seeing, hearing, feeling, thinking, changing our minds and so on and the concepts of neural activity belong to different categories, and as we shall see there are strong logical as well as other reasons against mixing them carelessly. But I suggest that we can have a duality without postulating a 'dualism' (in the sense of two 'worlds' and some kind of interaction).

If you want a label for what I'm going to suggest, you could call it 'comprehensive realism'. 'Realism' implies that we reckon with what must be *reckoned with*. We first and foremost reckon with the data of our conscious experience. Then secondly, we reckon, as obediently as we can, with the physical data (which we learn of through our conscious experience) about our brains. The adjective 'comprehensive' is meant to suggest an intellectual posture which insists on *confronting* those two things. Not pushing them into two water-tight compartments, but confronting, correlating, doing all we can to see where they fit together, comprehending them, holding them together and recognizing in this the unity of the cognitive agent that each of us is.

I believe that the interactionist and the materialist are each seeking to conserve a real truth about our human nature. The materialist recognizes that our physical embodiment invites (and rewards) analysis in the same physical terms as the rest of the material world. The interactionist recognizes that the reality of what it is to be a conscious agent is richer – has more to it – than can be described in material (or for that matter in mental) terms alone. What I wish to put forward is an option which can do justice to what mechanistic materialism and Cartesian interactionism are respectively trying to conserve, without their negative implications.

Embodiment of conscious agency

I wish to suggest, in other words, that we try, as a philosophical way through our subject, the idea that our conscious experience is *embodied in* our brain activity (rather than interacting with it from another world, or being identical with it in a sense that would be reductionist in its outcome). As against the identity theorists, who would say that mental events are just brain events renamed, I would suggest that we try out the philosophical hypothesis that mental events and brain events are two complementary aspects of conscious human agency.

The central concept is conscious human agency. It is, after all, our primary ground (rather than 'matter' or 'mind', both of which are heavily theory-laden abstractions from the data of our experience). If, metaphorically speaking, you make a projection of this concept onto the outside world, then you derive an image of brain events; if instead, you take the standpoint of the agent himself, then you experience mental events – conscious experience. The two are related in the way that complementary descriptions in geometry are related. In the case of the plan and elevation drawings of a house, for example, it would be silly to say that the plan drawing is 'nothing but' and identical with the elevation drawing, and yet they are both projections of one and the same house which has more dimensions – more degrees of freedom conceptually – than plan or elevation alone.

Efficacy – but not causality

I would suggest along these lines that we can expect to find an inter-dependence between mental activity and brain activity. This is, we note in passing, an interdependence without *interference* of the sort that interactionism would postulate – without any of what Roger Sperry in his philosophy has called 'pushing and hauling'. He has talked about the mind as acting on the brain, 'pushing and hauling the system around'. I suggest that we don't need to go to that extreme: if one is embodied in the other then the interdependence is, in a sense, *closer* than if one were pushing and hauling on the other.

Yet I would insist along these lines on the *determinative efficacy* of our thinking, valuing, choosing and so forth. Just as – to use the analogy to which I referred earlier – the weather predicting programs embodied in a computer determine, for the time being, the behaviour of the computer, so our thinking and valuing determine our behaviour – efficaciously – at least from time to time.

I prefer not to call the link 'causal' because normally we use the term cause or causality to point to relations of dependence within one conceptual level – one physical force causing another force, or one information flow causing another information flow. But the relation now is between the two levels and I think if we call the relationship one of *interdependence* it will be less misleading.

Summary: the conscious control of action

[*What, then, are brains for? One might want to say that first and foremost the brain is the organ of our conscious agency and experience. Certainly one can safely say that our brains are for handling information. One can see brains as the embodiment of our information-processing activities, so that brains stand to these activities somewhat as 'hardware' stands to the running of the 'software' in a computer.*

Of particular interest among these activities are those which we would describe as intelligent human agency.] In this chapter we have been thinking about the essential ingredients of agency which we would regard as intelligent, and we identified two functions of a 'supervisory' nature. The first was the determination of current goals and the running assessment and ordering of priorities. The second (which will be further explored in the next two chapters) is the updating of the internal repertoire of 'conditional readinesses' for action and the planning of action, in matching response to the demands of sensory input. Each of these is a function that could be expected to have a correlate in conscious experience; the first under such headings as decision or volition, the second under the heading of perception (as distinct from mere sensorimotor coordination, which can take place subconsciously). (This paragraph is taken from MacKay, 1980a).

Notes

1 [*The gun's final position – its bearing and elevation – is one implicit representation of its target's (predicted) position. It is instructive to note that there may not need to be, at any earlier stage of the calculations, a unitary representation of a target's three coordinates.*]

2 For a fuller appraisal of the experimental evidence which Eccles sees as pointing to the external influence of the mind on the brain, see MacKay (1982a).

4

Perception

I think it may be helpful to set the scene by saying a few things about the question of perception in general. Having come into the field as a physicist myself, some 35 years ago, I can well remember some of the stumbling blocks past which I had to trip; and I think it may be good to keep a few points in mind as landmarks. You will then be much less likely to try to understand the perceptual system, as many of us did when we came fresh to brain research, as some kind of 'input–throughput–output' transmitting system.

The central notion that focuses thinking about living organisms, for this purpose, is the notion of *agency*. What is characteristic about a living organism is that it *acts in view of ends*, and that it matches itself to its world by way of a sensory system. We have to think of the brain, then, not merely as a physical system, nor merely as a physiological, biochemical system, but also as an *organization*. The image of an organization (for example, a human organization) has to be kept in our minds all the time, as well as images appropriate to the physical systems which we know of course to exist in the brain.

There are many sorts of organization we can consider by way of corrective to over-simple notions about the brain. Think of a sales organization, a military organization, a relief organization, for example. The central notion in all of these is that of a repertoire of action. This repertoire has to be used in a world which has a certain structure, certain regular, predictable features; and the problem for the organism from this formal point of view is that of selecting from the repertoire (we spoke of subroutines for feeding, fight and flight, and there are learned subroutines too) in such a way as to further the ends of the organism in the world. The organizing system, O, can be thought of as embodying these subroutines and determining implicitly the probabilities that, in given circumstances, *if* the organism wants to do a particular thing, *if* the goal is such and such, *then* a particular course of action will be chosen.

Updating

Vision, together with the other senses, has from this point of view the function of enabling such things as locomotor action to take place efficiently, so that obstacles are avoided, prey is identified and pounced on successfully, and so forth. The sensory systems can be regarded as a surface which is in contact with the world from which signals impinge, this surface's function being to bring up to date the organization of the selective process in the repertoire.

[*The process by which a system such as that of figure 3.2 could use the signals from the receptors to build up within its organizing system, O, an internal representation of the stable features of the world against which the system is struggling, will be dealt with in later chapters. Let us consider, for the moment, the* nature *of this internal information store that is to be updated.*]

Not a 'map', but a readiness for action in the world

To spell out the sort of thing I mean, let us take a very simple example. Suppose you drive your car up a semi-circular drive into its garage. In the garage the front wheels will be at a certain angle to the chassis. This angle of the wheels *implicitly represents* the curvature of the drive. It has set up in the car what you could call, in an obvious sense, a 'state of conditional readiness': the car is 'conditionally ready' to follow the required path if and when it is set in motion. Even though nothing happens for weeks, if you were to drive the car backwards (we neglect friction and various other complications) then the car would follow more or less the curvature of the drive. So the setting of the wheel implicitly represents the curvature of the drive in view of the goal of following the path of the drive. If it were not that the car (or car plus driver) had a goal of following the drive, the angle of the wheels wouldn't represent anything. But given that this is a goal-directed system, the angle of the wheels represents a 'conditional readiness' to match the shape of the drive. You don't need to have a little picture of the drive inside the car for this purpose, all you need is the appropriate constraint on its repertoire of action.

That is the simplest example I can think of and you can just imagine how much more complicated must be the conditional readiness of a person playing a game of chess or engaging in conversation. But if you'll allow the thing as an illustration, what I am now suggesting is that we think of the brain as embodying within its elaborate structure – which has, you remember, millions of fibres intersecting with millions of fibres to give rise to a variety of probabilities that in certain circumstances such and such will happen and so on – a state of conditional readiness to match the world as that particular organism has encountered it in and through its sensory and other activities.

Representation of the external world

Along these lines, we are coming to the idea that your world of action could be represented in the information system of your brain not by a little model in any literal topographic sense, or a little picture, but by an immensely complex 'conditional probability network'. (I know these are jargon words but I hope you get the flavour of them.) In the case of our motor car it is in a state where nothing need happen but it is in a state of 'conditional readiness', such that *if* it is driven backwards then there is a high probability that it will follow the curvature of the drive. In that general sense we can think of the external world (your external world and mine) as represented in the information network of your brain by the state of conditional readiness, which in principle could be summed up in millions and millions of probability statements of the form: if this were the goal and that were the environment (for example, if he wanted to put bacon and eggs on and he were at home) then he would be conditionally ready to turn this way, open the refrigerator and so on. That sort of statement would be one of millions and millions to which the current hook-up in the brain would be equivalent.

This then is a theory of the way the hook-up for activity in the world can come to function as a representation of the features of the world. If you want an illustration of a 'hook-up' whose complexity lies between that of the brain and that of our simple steering wheel, think of the conditional readiness represented by the lever settings in a railway shunting yard. There are dozens, or these days hundreds, of levers which set up a conditional readiness. Nothing need be happening at the moment, but *if* a particular set of trucks comes along a particular track then signals will be set to red here and green there and the points to such and such positions. So the lever and other settings are determining the probabilities that in stated circumstances – that is why I call them *conditional* probabilities – this condition will lead to that action.

In this sense our flow-map of figure 3.2 points to the organizing system as the general location of the representation of the perceptual world. Our image of the perceived world is implicitly embodied in our state of organization to cope with it.

Perception: an outwardly directed matching response

I would like us to consider the possibility that perception is represented, in information flow terms, as the updating (the bringing up to date and keeping up to date) of the state of conditional readiness of the organizing system, O, to match the demands coming in through the sensory system. What correlates directly with our conscious experience in perceiving (i.e. with what we actually perceive as distinct from all the information that bombards our sensory surface) is an internal matching response.

Perception is a response, a matching response, I suggest, to the demands of sensory input. This is important: the theory of perception has got itself, in the past, into several tangles through failing to distinguish between, on the one hand, the reception and processing of the sensory input and, on the other hand, perceiving.

Reception and sensory analysis is an inwardly flowing informational activity – from the receptors in, consisting of filtering and so forth and represented by the box in figure 3.2 called feedforward, FF. This teases out the information: we talked about Hubel–Wiesel cells doing that in chapter 2. Our model assumes the existence of banks of such filters in the input to the organizing system, permitting a preliminary extraction of cues to which the internal organizing system then has to match itself. So reception happens in parallel, many-fold, million-fold.

Perceiving, on the other hand, is a unitary process in matching response to the multiple parallel demands of the sensory input.

In terms of this information-flow model the region of *attention* (attention being as it were the focus of perception) would be the region currently under active matching. By this I mean the region of the visual or other field currently under active matching in the sense that the supervisory system is bringing up to date the conditional readiness to reckon with it, and nothing else, at the moment.

The diagram of figure 3.2, then, has in it room enough for some crucial distinctions in the theory of perception. There is the distinction between sensation and perception (or sensory demand and perception) and also the distinction between that to which attention is paid and that to which it is not. Distinctions between focal and subsidiary attention can also be drawn.

The unity of our perceptual world

I think the best way to make this clear will be to apply it to some examples. Take first the case of tactile perception. Suppose you wake up in the night and you don't want to put the light on, so you use your hands to fumble on the bedside table to find your handkerchief. What do you do? Of course you allow both surfaces (why use only one hand!) to roam around as quickly as possible and eventually one of them comes on what you are 'looking for'. How come you don't feel two tactile worlds because you have, after all, put two receptor surfaces around? And you say to me, don't be silly, why should I? There is only one world for me; that is the world in which I have to *act*. It is the 'domain of action' that defines my world. What my sensory surfaces do is to make demands on me to get ready for it, to cope with it. The unity of my world of the bedside table is the unity of my field of action and the multiplicity of my sensory surfaces is neither here nor there.

This may sound so obvious as to be ridiculous and you may wonder why I say it. The reason is that in the case of vision, oddly enough, the

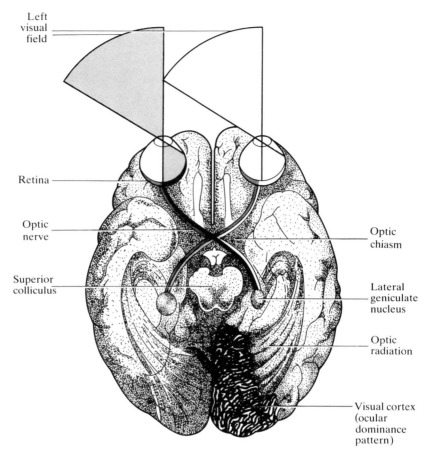

Left
visual
field

Retina

Optic
nerve

Superior
colliculus

Optic
chiasm

Lateral
geniculate
nucleus

Optic
radiation

Visual cortex
(ocular
dominance
pattern)

Figure 4.1   Diagram of paths from the retinae to the cortex at the rear of the head. From each eye the left half of the visual field is projected to the right occipital region of the brain (and the right half visual field to the left brain). Within the ocular dominance bands the majority of cells are responsive to signals from both eyes; there is not an abrupt switch from left to right eye, but a smooth transition with contributions from the two eyes represented in gradually altering proportions.

same point has not been taken at all. Let us move to the case of vision: this time in exploring for the handkerchief we 'throw our eye around the room'. What we mean is that we use our eye muscles to throw around the room the particular patch which optically projects from our retina. So the retina, optically projected out through the lens and

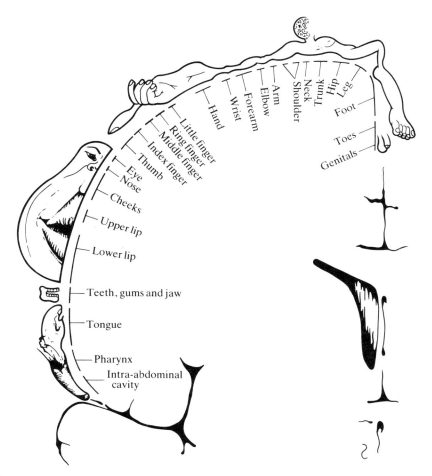

Figure 4.2 Mapping of the body surface on to the post central gyrus (a strip of cortex over the crown of head above the ears) as determined by electrical stimulation of the cortex in waking patients. The relative sizes of the bodily parts represent the area of cortex allocated to them. It will be noted that the hand shown is the right hand, because this is the left half cortex. Its movements are also largely controlled from (a neighbouring region of) the left cortex. The left half of the body is mapped symmetrically on to the right cortex. (Penfield and Rasmussen, 1950.)

onto some part of the field, is not unlike the palm of your hand from this point of view. Throwing your eye around the room is logically analogous to throwing your palm around the room. As a result your sensitive surface, the retina, is subject to demands which you experience as sights, and these demands set up in you a conditional readiness to reckon with different parts of your world.

Now of course in the case of your eye there isn't just one little sensory surface, there are millions of receptors and furthermore, as we can see in figure 4.1, the sensory surface is represented on the two halves of the rear of our brains.

[*The situation in the case of the hands, however, is not in principle different.*] Figure 4.2 shows where in the brain the information from the right hand is processed. [*The information from the left hand is processed in the symmetrical region of the other hemisphere (not shown).*] So these brain areas are individual to each hand. As can be seen from the cartoons around the edge of the brain, each hand and each side of the body has its signals processed largely on the other side of the brain.

This general pattern also prevails for the visual system: the projection from each *half* of the retina in each eye-ball projects to one half brain so that the left half of our field of view is processed in the right half of the head and the right half of the field of view in the left side of the head. So we have got two visual 'maps'. And there has been no end of argument in the past as to how we see one world, with no detectable 'seam' up the middle, when the map of the visual world is split into two on the back of our head. What I'm suggesting is that by starting from thinking about tactile exploration we dissolve pseudo-mysteries of this sort. There is no mystery here because there is not a problem. The split processing of the demands from the left and right half of the retina is on the same footing as the split processing of the demands from the left and right hands. All that matters is that we have one repertoire of action. This repertoire of action in the world is shaped in its conditional readiness by the visual and by the tactile demand.

Well, you say, we have got two eyes and that's a further problem, and certainly if you cross your eyes you do seem to see two worlds. That is indeed a special difficulty of the visual system because the system has developed to gain a lot of information about depth and other things by superimposing the two images. So it is not surprising that you get in trouble when you use a trick involving convergence and focusing, which the two eyes have developed to see through brushwood and so on, and which the palms don't have.[1] But the logical point, that the mere diversity and multiplicity of so-called 'maps' of the sensory area within the head does not have any tendency to create a multiplicity and diversity of perceived worlds, applies just as much in the case of vision as in that of touch. The visual world is one for the same reason that the tactile world is one: there is a single action space and *a single state of conditional readiness for action in it*.

What I am suggesting is that we look for the physical correlates of perceiving not in the *receptive* area of the brain, but rather in the organizing system which prepares and maintains the 'conditional readiness' of the organism for the state of affairs giving rise to the received signals. On this basis to perceive something (say an object in one's path) is to respond by internal adaptation to it (setting up conditional readinesses to avoid it, grasp it, describe it, etc. in case of need); and the unity or 'wholeness' of an object as perceived reflects the integration of the 'state of conditional readiness' to match the stimuli from it.

The stability of the perceived world

We have been talking so far about the unity of the perceived world. The same point [*(that our state of organization for action is the key to thinking about perception)*] applies to its stability. In the case of tactile exploration you rub your palm around the table by your bed and of course you experience rubbing sensations; there is relative movement between your exploring surface and the thing you're exploring. Why doesn't the explored surface appear to be moving about? Well, it never occurs to us to ask that. If each finger tip of an exploring hand signals 'rubbing' of about equal velocity this indicates the presence of an extended rigid surface, and if the velocity comes within the range we anticipate from the hand movement we made, then we are satisfied that the surface is at rest. Similarly in the visual case, if you throw your eye around the room, then the retinal image is moving over your retina – but there's been no end of argument as to why we don't see the world as swinging around us when we move our eyes voluntarily from A to B. Logically there's no more reason to make a fuss about the one case than the other. What you are doing in planting your projected retina on different parts of the world is sampling the demands made, in this case optically, by different parts of your world on your conditional readiness – in the same way as you would with your palm if you had the chance.

[*The 'problem' of the stability of the visual world has been felt to be highlighted by the following observation, which goes back to Aristotle.*] When I move my line of gaze voluntarily from left to right, I get little or no impression that the world is moving, although the visual image dances across my retina. When, however, I move the line of gaze through the same angle by pressing on the corner of the open eyelid, so softly as to rule out any possibility of mechanical distortion of the eyeball, I perceive violent movement of the visual field from right to left. This has led to elaborate theories of 'cancellation' of the shifts of the retinal image, implying that in the voluntary case there must be some neural discharge which in effect moves the optical image backwards by the amount by which it was voluntarily displaced. A cancellation mechanism of this sort *is* often used to preserve a 'true north' map on a radar display, where, of course, there is an operator witnessing on a screen an image of the external world. That kind of thinking is called for in the case of television too, where indeed motion of the image is a problem: if you swing a television camera, then on the receiving screen everything sweeps around. But there is no evidence that there is a 'receiving screen' in that sense inside the head.

[*The lecture proceeded from here to the start of the next chapter. The lecture notes, however, suggest that some further points were intended for the book. The remainder of this chapter is derived from Donald MacKay's writings to fulfil this intention and permit the interested reader to see at greater length what MacKay's updating view of perception entails.*]

Visual stability

The 'explanation' that has often been offered for the above facts is that in the case of a voluntary eye movement the innervation of oculomotor muscles provides 'compensation' which is absent when rotation of the eyeball is due to other causes, such as the external finger. This is rather vague and suffices only to raise further questions. *How* does innervation of eye muscles result in such accurate compensation for the retinal image displacement? Is it done by pre-computation on the basis of the outgoing oculomotor stimuli (the 'outflow' theory)? If so it relies with remarkable success on the transfer characteristics (the input-output relations) of the oculomotor system. Is it done by post-computation on the basis of proprioceptive stimuli from the oculomotor muscles (the 'inflow' theory)? This is perhaps one way in which a designer of automata would solve the problem. It exchanges uncertainty as to the transfer characteristics of the oculomotor system, for uncertainty as to those of the proprioceptors, which might well be more stable – if in fact there were proprioceptors of adequate accuracy in the right places and in adequate numbers. But are there? In the goat Whitteridge has found some, and in man they have been reported, but with little evidence of the anatomical connections, and still less of accuracy of the sort required by a 'compensation' theory. Clearly this would be a shaky hypothesis on which to base a general theory of the observed stability of the visual world – although I confess that for a time I could think of no better.

In fact there is another possibility, which takes us a stage further back. We have so far been considering the voluntary eye movement as a *fait accompli*: something that has happened for reasons of its own, with certain unfortunate consequences for the retinal image which we must now annul as best we can. Suppose, however, that we ask how – in what circumstances and in what way – the voluntary movement itself comes about. When do I move my eye voluntarily? When I want to look elsewhere. How do I judge the movement is satisfactory? *By the change that has taken place in the retinal image.*

Here surely is the key to our problem. The change in the retinal image under voluntary movement is not merely a *consequence* of the movement: it is its *goal*. The stability of the visual field under voluntary movement is not a *deduction* from cues, but a *presupposition* or null-hypothesis on which the voluntary movement is based. There would, therefore, seem to be no reason to expect that the visual motion signals should be cancelled or suppressed. What is necessary is rather that the flow of information from the eye-movement system should modify the criteria of *evaluation* of these signals so that they become indications of the stability of the visual world rather than the contrary.

A number of simple demonstrations help, I think, to support this view of the matter. If we close one eye and press very lightly on the open eyelid at the corner, the visual world appears, as we have already said, to move. The impression of motion is irresistible. If we look closely, however, we find that the region around the fixation point appears to move *more* than the peripheral region; and in fact with very small movements we may not feel that the periphery is moving at all, but only the region around the fixation point. If we now do the same

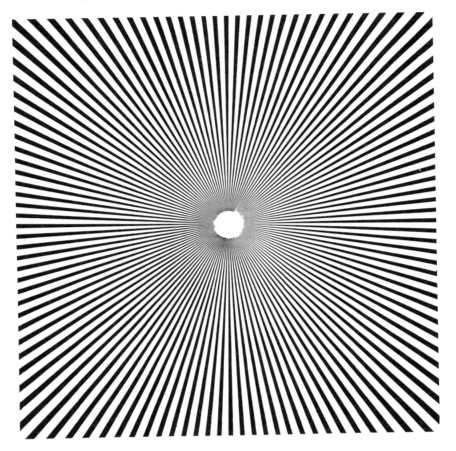

Figure 4.3 Ray figure.

while viewing figure 4.3, an interesting feature emerges. In addition to the displacement of the centre, we see a sort of 'rubber sheet' distension and contraction of the field, perpendicular to the direction of motion. For example, if the image is displaced from left to right, the regions at '3 o'clock' and '9 o'clock' seem to perform a fanwise expansion or contraction. Suppose finally that a vertical marker of some sort is introduced halfway along, say, the '3 o'clock' ray. At once the rubbery expansion in its vicinity ceases, although in the symmetrical region at 9 o'clock (without a marker) it is still present.

In each case what we see, I suggest, can be interpreted as the result of a mismatch of the evaluatory criteria: but these anomalies illustrate the thesis that our internal representation of the world is affected only in proportion as there is *information* to justify a change. On this principle, it is not surprising that when the visual image is displaced, we normally see the central region, which stimulates an area rich in detectors, as 'moving' more than the periphery. Again, in the absence of significant mismatch of a particular feature of the visual representation, no change in that feature is perceived. We do not see a displacement of figure 4.3 as a whole, because the translation of a contour along itself gives no information; but we do perceive an expansion corresponding to any change in separation of the contours. On the other hand, given a marker in the orthogonal direction, we see displacement but no expansion.

Let me mention a further striking illustration. If a small steadily glowing lamp is viewed against a background lit stroboscopically at about five flashes per second, and the same gentle eyeball pressing is repeated, a dramatic dissociation takes place (MacKay, 1958). With sufficiently gentle displacements, the lamp is seen to move, although the background remains stationary; yet the lamp is not seen to move relative to the background! Once again the change perceived is the minimum justified by the optical evidence, however *intellectually* improbable or absurd the change may be.

Perceptual constancy

[*A similar analysis shows that for such perceptual phenomena as the constancy of perceived sizes of objects during relative distance changes it is logically unnecessary to postulate any 'zoom lens' mechanism in the visual pathway.*]

The 'zoom' lens analogy

We humans perceive approaching or receding objects as constant in size even when their retinal size grows or diminishes. An automatic text reading device is normally designed to give the same output for a given input regardless of its size. It has seemed natural to many people to regard these performances by humans and machines as analogous, and various kinds of scale-changing mechanisms have been postulated to account for size constancy in human vision.

Object perception, not image perception

This analogy blurs a fundamental distinction between perceiving a
visual image on the one hand and perceiving the object giving rise to it
on the other: a distinction which has been greatly clarified by the work
of J. J. Gibson. (Plate 15 shows an example in which object perception so dominates image perception that we have the greatest difficulty
in recognizing the two images as the same.) To perceive an object is to
be conditionally ready to reckon with it in a great variety of ways other
than by giving it the correct name: by grasping it, walking around it
and so forth. These conditional readinesses are some of the operational implications of perceiving its size: and just as it requires information to set them up, so it requires information to change them. If an
object is approaching us or vice versa, the question to be settled by our
cerebral information system is not how to get rid of the change in size
of the retinal image, but how to do informational justice to it at the
level of our internal state of readiness which implicitly represents the
object. In particular, does the change supply information *incompatible*
with our previous readiness-for-the-size of the object?

Informational inertia

Constancy of the perceived world is a matter not of compensatory
distortion, but of informational evaluation of the sensory input. What
we have suggested so far is that perception in living organisms differs
from most 'artificial pattern recognition' in having as its end-product
an internal representation of the perceived *world* rather than of the
sensory *field* presented to the receptors. We could call this a 'matching
model', in the sense not of a neural replica, but rather of a generative
organizing system that maintains an appropriate state-of-conditional-
readiness-to-reckon-with the world as perceived. On this basis spatial
constancy (under transformations of sensory input caused by changes
in spatial relationship to particular objects) would be the natural
result of 'informational inertia' in the organizing system; for if these
transformations were completely matched by corresponding locational
changes in the 'model', there would be no residual error-information
to disturb the 'null-hypothesis' that the objects themselves are stable.
In other words the question asked by such a system is how par-

simoniously the 'model' can be altered to match the sensory demands. (This of course is an embodiment of the hypothetico-inductive method of science itself.)

Although this principle embodies a hypothesis, it can be supported on grounds of informational economy. Since the function of perception is to keep up to date the total organizing system, there would be 100 per cent redundancy between this updating activity and the contents of any internal display. It thus seems natural to ask whether the updating system itself could not serve to represent, implicitly, the world to which it adapts, so eliminating the redundancy. On this basis, the world would be internally represented in terms of the pattern of demand (actual or conditional) which it imposes on the perceiver (MacKay, 1956, 1962, 1965a).

The blind spot and scotomata

The idea that what we perceive is only what demands matching response makes sense of a number of further perceptual phenomena that at first sight have little in common. Consider first what is generally called the 'completion' of the visual scene across the receptor-free blind spot of the eye. [*This is the small circular region devoid of light receptors where the cabling of the optic nerve leaves from near the middle of the retina.*] Why do we not see our blind spot as a gap in the picture? By now we have a standard question to ask in response: what *demands* does the blind spot make on the supervisory system? Seeing-a-gap, like seeing anything else, requires a corresponding inflow of information sufficient to disturb the equilibrium state of the supervisory system. But the blind spot, having no receptors, generates no disturbance at all. Hence whatever the internal representation of the visual world may be, nothing discordant with it is contributed by the blind spot. It is rather as when we explore an object with our finger tips. Nothing discordant with the percept we form is contributed by the gaps between our fingers! Of course if we direct our blind spot steadily towards a small enough object (such as a person's head, or one's finger tip waggled at arm's length), then the absence of the expected visual signals can generate a significant mismatch, and we notice that the object is missing from view; but except in these special cases our blind spot does nothing to invalidate the 'null-hypothesis' based on our previous exploration of the scene. [*To locate your blind spot: close one eye and gaze at an object on the same level as your open eye; hold out the corresponding hand at the same horizontal level about two hands' widths from the fixated object on the side away from your nose and waggle the outer digit.*]

The same analysis applies to the 'completion' frequently observed across visual scotomata of cortical origin (see Teuber et al., 1960). [*Some victims of gunshot wounds or other damage at the back of the head may have only limited sectors of their visual field remaining in which they are able to detect the waggled finger or a flashed light. Nevertheless in everyday life they see the scene whole, though somewhat blurred in the direction of their scotoma.*] There is no need to account for this by imagining some cerebral synthesizer generating the missing parts of the picture; for in informational terms a missing cortical area contributes no evidence of mismatch.

By contrast, scotomata of retinal origin could be expected to be more frequently visible, since lesioned areas of retina (unlike the blind spot) have corresponding cortical receptive areas which are likely to be left in an abnormal state, and so to generate information discordant with the null-hypothesis.

What these examples illustrate may be termed the 'principle of informational parsimony': under normal circumstances, information is required to justify every distinctive feature in a situation-as-perceived.

Noticing things that are missing

We have so far spoken as if pattern recognition were always a matter of extracting relations between *data*. This, however, is too simple – or at least it overlooks a subtlety in the concept of a datum. The trouble is that in many cases (clinical syndromes, for example) the *absence* of a particular element may form a crucial feature of the pattern to be recognized. This may seem trivial. Cannot the absence of an element be just as much a datum as its presence? Indeed it can: but only when it has *occurred* to us that it might have been there.

Take, for instance, the case of an empty sky. What are the elements whose absence constitutes data? Aeroplanes? Clouds? Elephants? Newspapers? ... To pretend that an empty sky offers 'data' in this sense is to say that it offers an infinity of data. But then we shall need an infinity of computer time to go through these 'data' looking for relations between them and others. For a mere 16×16 elements of computer screen and only two states for the luminance of each element the number of 'negative data' is of the order of the number of particles in the Einstein universe. Mere quantization is laughably inadequate as a solution.

How then do we human beings cope with this situation when we recognize patterns that include negative data? Subjectively we say we were struck by the absence of something. 'I noticed that he didn't shake hands', or 'I was struck by the fact that he never smiled'. There must have been an infinity of other possibilities by whose absence we were not struck. Why, then, were we struck by these?

The answer, presumably, is that we brought our internal matching response system to the situation in a prepared state, set up with a generative model that would have matched the absent feature. Strictly speaking, it is not the absence of the feature but the presence of the mismatch signal that constitutes the datum.

This trite observation helps to bring out one further advantage of the active hypothetico-deductive matching approach in pattern recognition. It converts a situation in which there is nothing to *claim the attention* of a pattern-recognizer, into a positive datum that does (rightly or wrongly) claim attention; but it does so without the desperate device of treating *every* absent feature as a datum. Pattern recognition can be regarded as a process by which most data come to be systematically ignored in favour of a small subset that satisfy certain criteria of recognition, and so have competitive advantage. The problem is that although for a communication engineer a non-event may have as much selective information content as an event, from a physical standpoint it lacks the energy of an event and so is at a competitive disadvantage. A hypothetical match-and-comparison process can be thought of as a selective way of giving a small subset of all the non-events a voice (a physical representation in terms of energy) in the energy-based competition for attention.

Once we start thinking along these lines we can see a particular advantage of filters that attenuate the relative physical strength of signals representing *redundant* claims. It is not simply that the energy per bit of information is thereby kept to a minimum. The point is that if recognition of patterns depends in part on an energy-based cerebral competition, it would make sense for the system to tend to equalize the physical advantage of signals of equal potential import for pattern formation. The wealth of contrast-enhancement, OFF- as well as ON-responsive units, adaptation, after-discharge and the like can all be seen in this light as providing better chances for certain classes of non-event to catch the attention of the pattern-sensitive system, and better balanced chances for typical events.

At levels of the nervous system where there is little or no element of competition, this argument does not apply, and there may be no advantage in representing a particular concept by the excitation of a single neuron rather than by a particular cooperative state of many simultaneous active elements.

The null-method of pattern recognition

[*Other illustrations could be given in support of the thesis above, that we carry in our brains a state of organization which matches itself continuously to the incoming data. Thus we form a clear view of a landscape glimpsed only fragmentarily through trees or other obstructions; we see moving objects as single objects in motion and not as a series of objects at different positions. The* exclusiveness *of perceptual interpretation is a further example mentioned below and tacit knowledge is the concern of chapter 11.*]

Of *tacit recognition* it may be remarked here: Perhaps the most significant feature of a null-method of pattern recognition from a philosophical standpoint is that it could enable a perfectly definite act of recognition to take place without necessarily enabling the recognizer to *specify* what features in the input were critical. In the limit, a mechanism could grope its way into a matching response without any preprocessing and feature classification of the input at all. Its only internal label for the input would be its generative matching-response configuration.

Profiting from redundancy

When we move our eyes or our bodies, or when other objects move, although there are myriads of changes in our sensory input, most of these changes happen together: they are not independent. As I look around a room full of stable objects, no change is taking place in the visual demand on my adaptive system. I may be inspecting different parts of it, but the correlation between successive samples is so high that the whole visual inflow represents a very small information rate.

In a relatively stable and structured environment the sensory input to an organism shows massive redundancy in the information-theoretic sense. Action in that environment, however elaborate and varied, can therefore be planned and steered largely on the basis of information already received and stored. From the standpoint of information engineering, perception is an adaptive exploitation of the redundancy in the pattern of demand imposed by the sensory input. The main form taken by this redundancy can be termed covariation.

Covariation

Most of us who work on the visual system are tempted to take vision as the paradigm case of perception; and when we think of vision we tend to think of our ability to recognize at a glimpse the form and disposition of objects in visual space. When I look at a triangle I have a triangular distribution of excited receptors on my retina. Here it may seem natural to suppose that the problem of perception would be solved if we could discover form-specific interactions between the simultaneously excited elements of the neural network, leading to a unique geometrical analysis of the figure of excitation.

When we turn to other modalities, however, the situation is strikingly different, even with spatial perception. To *feel* an object is not in general to have a topographic image of it on the receptors. Try, for example, the experiment of feeling a coat button with a finger tip or a finger nail. One perceives vividly the shape and details of the surface without a trace of topographic similarity between the sensory figure of excitation and the shape perceived. We have no difficulty in forming, as we say, a 'mental image' of the shapes and layout of suitable objects within range of our exploring fingers. In the case of the single finger nail, this is done without benefit of any somato-sensory 'feature detectors' analogous to those found in the visual system. The same holds for a blind man's perception of the road surface as he explores, for example, a manhole cover with his cane. The features are clearly perceived at the tip of the cane, although the only sensory input comes from the controlling hand and arm. The information is generated from the way in which *sensory inputs covary with exploratory action*, and from the way one sensory input covaries with another as exploration proceeds. Since the incoming signals do not form any 'neural image' in a topographic sense, the tactile world can only be represented *implicitly* by the way in which the sensory signals from fingers and proprioceptors covary with the exploratory motor-activity.

Still more remarkably, many blind people are able to perceive an obstacle, such as a closed door in their path, without tactile contact. To them it feels as if the door 'presses' or 'radiates' on their cheeks, and they call their perceptual capacity 'facial vision'; but it turns out that this disappears if their ears are blocked! The physical basis here is in fact acoustic interference between the ambient sounds entering the ear directly and after reflection from the obstacle. Here it is the covariation of the acoustic spectrum with the movements of the subject that mediates perception of its direction and distance. Covariations of tactile, auditory, visual and other sensory inputs are normal concomitants of most action, and must be presumed to provide most of our normal clues for the integrated perception of our environment.

The detection and analysis of covariation is thus the main function required of the relevant cortical network. Given this, the system has all it needs by way of an internal representation of the tactile world-as-perceived for the organization of relevant action. The state of conditional readiness for action using other dimensions of the effector system, such as walking, can be derived directly from this representation, without any need for an explicit 'map'.

Probing

The above examples may be sufficient to suggest that in considering the neurophysiological correlates of perception in general we might miss some essential insights if we were to take visual pattern recognition as paradigmatic. In pursuit of this theme it is mentally loosening to try the converse approach, considering spatial perception as normally involving *probing* of an agent's environment. Vision is then approached as a special case of probing with elaborate feedforward.

At first glance the concept of probing might seem to have little to do with visual perception. As a probe the retina is exquisitely equipped to take in an extensive topographic sample of the visual field at each fixation. The visual nervous system is replete with cells that respond preferentially to local geon.etrical features of the retinal image, suggesting that pattern analysis of the figure of sensory excitation here plays a role not paralleled in an exploratory probing with a finger nail. It is well known, moreover, that a single photoflash-lit sample of an unfamiliar scene can generate a positive after-image, lasting many seconds, in which a surprising amount of fine detail can be picked out without benefit of exploratory eye-movements or other sensory probing. Any suggestion that spatial vision *requires* ocular exploration is thus untenable.

On the other hand, it is equally undeniable that in normal vision exploratory eye-movements play a crucial part. The motor system used in visual probing of the environment comprises the whole muscular apparatus as it affects head position, as well as the oculomotor system. Admittedly, various reflexes allow the orientation of the eyes to be stabilized against certain head movements; but as Gibson points out, even when moving through a textured world with constant head- and eye-orientation, we receive a succession of visual signals that covary with locomotion so as to provide information both about our own motion and about the layout-in-depth of surfaces around us (Gibson, 1950).

This suggests that we ask what kind of cross-correlation might usefully be computed between the signals from an extended array of retinal receptors, both in relation to one another and in relation to motor activity. Reichardt (1957), in a pioneering analysis, has shown the importance of auto-correlation as a functioning principle of the central nervous system, and has investigated in detail some computing operations required for visual tracking by insects. Taking hints from the psychophysical work of Gibson and others, we might expect to find that computations are performed of such features as local optical texture density and its gradients in space and time, the velocity of image drift and its gradients, and thus the covariation (if any) of signals originating in a group of neighbouring receptors (indicating the presence of an optically rigid extended surface). These computations would be additional to any involved in geometrical pattern analysis and would serve mainly to provide clues as to the disposition-in-space of objects around the head and of its motion relative to them. Covari-

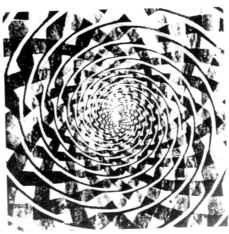

Figure 4.4   The Fraser spiral. The twisted cords all lie on concentric circles (Fraser, 1908.)

ation of these features with motor activity would then be particularly informative, leading to an internal representation of the world just as in other forms of sensory probing.

How then might the diverse functions of passive image analysis and active probing be integrated? If a major goal of the perceptual system is to get the external world represented in the form of conditional instructions for reckoning with it, it seems a natural hypothesis that both image-analysis and visual probing-with-cross-correlation contribute feedforward to shape different aspects of the matching strategy of the supervisory system, SS. (The first might be more closely related to the 'what' of perception, and the second to the 'where' – in line perhaps with the growing evidence of the different contributions of the geniculo-striate and tectal subsystems of the brain to visual perception.)

Visual perception in reality covers a continuous spectrum of experience from the almost wholly passive to the consciously active. One extreme is illustrated by the well-known optical illusion of figure 4.4, where specially designed local geometrical features generate feedforward so compelling that no amount of active intellectual effort can prevent a non-veridical matching-response at a superficial level. The perception of spirality is irresistible; yet the twisted cords are all in fact circular. At the opposite extreme stand the perceptual puzzles

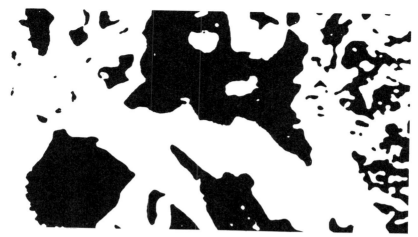

Figure 4.5   The hidden man. (Porter, 1954.)

such as figure 4.5, where the seeing of the 'hidden' face is a skill demanding conscious effort of a hypothesis-testing kind. In between come most cases of normal perception, where we may suppose that 'passive' feedforward from image-feature analysis constrains the active matching strategy of the supervisory system to produce a more or less veridical conditional readiness with a minimum of trial-and-error. There is some suggestion in the psychophysical literature that the supervisory activity may include 'tuning' the passive analysers to the perceptual task in hand (e.g. Jonides and Gleitman, 1972; Potter, 1954; Carr and Bacharach, 1976).

From this standpoint, there seems no necessary antithesis between two currently contrasted views of visual perception. On the one hand, authors such as R. L. Gregory have stressed the geometrical ambiguity inherent in two-dimensional retinal images of three-dimensional objects, and suggested that perception must depend on the construction and testing of *hypotheses* to fit the sensory data, on the basis of stored accessory knowledge. Against this, J. J. Gibson and his school consider the additional clues to three-dimensionality available in texture-gradients and the like to be normally sufficient to specify three-dimensional percepts uniquely, even without binocular stereopsis. On the view here recommended, these processes are not alternatives; the second can well serve as feedforward for the first. With sufficient feedforward the matching response can be uniquely determined; but

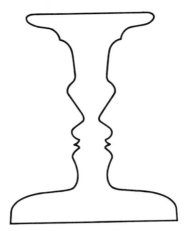

Figure 4.6   Candlestick and faces.

with an impoverished input the process would shade over into hypothetical trial-and-error. Where figures are ambiguous (see below) this
would lead to alternations between rival matching responses, subjectively experienced as perceptual rivalry.

The exclusiveness of perception

We have seen that there are several features of human pattern-
perception which invite interpretation in terms of an internal matching or nulling process. But perhaps one of the chief is the *exclusiveness*
of perceptual interpretation.

So far, we have tended to speak as if one internal matching response
were necessary and sufficient for any given stimulus configuration,
but there are many cases in which this is clearly not so. The well-
known ambiguous drawing of figure 4.6 can be seen *either* as a pair of
faces *or* as a candlestick, perhaps in rapid alternation, but not as both
at the same time. Each can be felt to 'exhaust' the drawing in its turn.
With a simple scanning filter or holographic pattern-detector, on the
other hand, all three figures (two faces and a candlestick) would be
signalled as simultaneously present. The same point emerges in relation to the familiar 'reversible' perspective drawings typified by figure
4.7, where a 'filtering-and-classifying' system would require *ad hoc*
machinery to prevent it from giving two output signals, whereas a

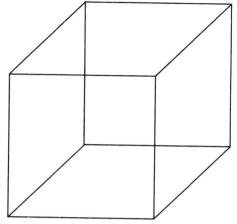

Figure 4.7 Necker cube.

'null' system could of course balance out the input in only one way at a time.

The contents of this page may be perceived equally accurately as ink on paper, as a succession of letters or as a succession of English sentences. In each case, the internal matching response is characteristically distinguished by the *class* of conditional readinesses associated with it. In our terms, 'seeing ... as' implies 'being ready to *reckon* with ... as'. When we are perceiving the contents of the page as an argument with which we disagree, it comes as something of a shock to be asked about the colour of granularity of the ink or the font of the letters. We may even need to look again; our current matching response had not been at a level that made us ready to reckon with these particular aspects of what lay before us. Our internal representation, although complete in itself, was in other terms – not inconsistent with, but complementary to, the terms required to do justice to those aspects now under discussion.

In the neural organization, such exclusiveness points to a *hierarchic* structure in the generator of perceptual matching responses. A response that matches a given visual or auditory input, for example, may be initiated at different levels in this hierarchy, and the criteria of 'match' or 'mismatch' may be set in correspondingly different terms. In principle there is no reason why matching responses should not take place simultaneously at different levels, but the evidence of subjective perception is that this is normally possible only at the expense of overall speed or accuracy. The more closely we try to follow changes at one level, the more the changes become exclusive of perception of details at other levels. The correlate in information-engineering terms would seem to be that the central evaluator of mismatch has a limited channel capacity, which must be shared between different levels, if more than one is to be 'attended to' at one time. The quality of perception is determined by the kind of internal activity called into being rather than by the configuration of sensory signals *per se*.

This last theme is dramatically illustrated by cases of ambiguity of perceived modality – in which the subject is mistaken as to which of his senses provides him with a particular percept. We mentioned above how totally blind people often feel they detect obstacles by what they call 'facial vision'. This feels to them as if it depended upon the skin of their faces; but experiment shows that they are relying on acoustic echoes of ambient noise. Only by making special efforts can they perceive the acoustical phenomena as such.

The exploring retinae

We began by reminding ourselves that the perceiving self is first and foremost an agent: the possessor of a repertoire of modes of *potential action* in his field. Action we distinguished from mere activity by the element of evaluation, which assesses the action as less or more satisfactory, attaching a match/mismatch value to it in the light of current criteria of evaluation. Fundamental to the approach here advocated is the principle whereby concepts are internally represented in an information system by *conditional instructions for (internal or external) action*.

For what sort of action should we expect the visual neural representation to maintain conditional readiness? First and foremost, I suggest, for ocular action – i.e. for action whereby the two retinae (as projected by the lenses) are enabled to dance around the visual world. Such action involves not only the oculomotor musculature, but all motor systems (of head, neck or limbs) that affect the ongoing selection of retinal samples of the environment. My suggestion is that the final central representation of the visual world is whatever neural configuration (in space and time) specifies the system's *conditional readiness for ocular navigation* in that world. To put it more generally, 'seeing' means first and foremost apprehending a complex of constraints on the planning of further 'looking' – constraints imposed by, and implicitly representative of, the structure of the world-as-seen. All the other consequences of seeing – our conditional readiness for moving our bodies around in our world, describing its contents, etc. – can readily be computed from the state of conditional readiness for ocular action.

We have of course to recognize the enormous disparity between the amount of geometrical information supplied by a single retinal sample (e.g. with flash illumination) and that supplied by a finger tip or even a whole hand. But the same general point applies. The covariation of retinal signals with ocular action is in principle an adequate source of information about the structure of the visual world. Moreover, even the rich structural-information content of a single retinal sample is all implicit in the spatio-temporal covariation of signals from different retinal locations. [*So we come back to the illustration with which we began this discussion of pattern vision on p. 83: the viewing of a triangle.*] If the oculomotor system is thought of as a means of moving the sampling retinae around the visual world, the primary function of the retinal array, in this context, is to supply *feedforward* for its exploratory programme.

The hypothesis that cortical neurones are primarily detectors of covariation offers a new way of looking at the functions of simple and complex cells. Instead of asking what elementary geometrical features of optical patterns (whether edges or spatial periodicities) a given cell 'detects', we should perhaps ask *what kinds of covariation* in the signals from the optical array it is equipped to sense.[2] Sensitivity to particular oriented edges and/or bars and/or gratings could well be important clues to the answer; but we might well miss the main functional point if we rested content with classifying and analysing cells solely in these terms. The experiments of Hammond and MacKay mentioned in chapter 2 show that there must be types of covariation more complex than those caused by these stimuli.

The otherwise puzzling multiplicity of visual areas would have a natural interpretation. As noted in chapter 2 there are several (in fact nowadays the number has gone up to about twenty) different 'visual areas' in the brain, some devoted to signalling motion, some signalling colour, some signalling orientation of lines and so on. The information from the eyes sprays out into many areas in parallel. What is going on is, so far as we know, never drawn back together into some little 'TV picture' somewhere else in the head. What it does is to funnel in on the state of conditional readiness to reckon with the world. To this end the diverse populations of 'feature-sensitive' cells in the various visual areas would serve not to delineate 'images' of different degrees of 'crudity', but rather to detect covariations of different degrees of generality, each of which can contribute directly to the total 'conditional probability matrix' that specifies the system's current grasp of its visual environment.

If the system has several different categories of covariation in which to 'listen out', it will be in the interests of signal-to-noise ratio to keep physically separate the associative networks seeking correlations in the different categories. Instead of looking for the anatomical basis of final integration in some 'superposition of maps in register', we should seek for it in (eventual) convergence from each area onto appropriate subdivisions of the system responsible for the conduct of ocular action. In that system (wherever it may be) the visual world-as-perceived would find itself represented not by a topographic 'map', but by a configuration of conditional readinesses adapted to take account of all its features in the planning of ocular action.

Vision with a stabilized image

At the other extreme from ocular exploration is the case of vision with a stabilized image. [*(Stabilization of the image on the retina may be achieved by the use of a contact lens bearing a stalk to which is attached a small mirror (Ditchburn, 1969).*] As is well-known, in this case the perceived image rapidly fades, but it can be revived either by slightly displacing or by modulating the brightness of the stabilized stimulus. Where a partially stabilized image of high contrast refuses to fade, it can, nevertheless, be 'wiped out' as a whole by moving over it an unstabilized image, which seems to give rise to a form of 'monocular rivalry'.

Now it is unlikely that simple physiological satiation can account for the fading of stabilized images. Although it doubtless plays a significant part, there is no evidence that such adaptation could be sufficient to abolish completely the primary cortical response to a stabilized image. Indeed anyone who has worked with conventional animal preparations must be familiar with cells in area 17 that respond tonically for many seconds to suitably patterned stimulation, even when (by virtue of curarization) the retinal image is fully stabilized.

Why then do no such patterns remain visible to human observers under complete image stabilization? The answer on our present hypothesis is clear. Stabilization, even if it does not abolish all retinal signals, eliminates all covariation. If no correlated changes take place, there is nothing for analysers of covariation to analyse. If, then, seeing depends on the results of covariational analysis, there will be no seeing. Furthermore, in the case where a poorly stabilized image generates a sufficiently fluctuating retinal output for analysers of covariation to work upon, the same hypothesis would predict that adding a strong background of coherently changing signals from an unstabilized image could readily saturate the population of covariance detectors, so as to swamp the feebler covariations in the poorly stabilized input, causing the original image to fade from view.

[*How then, in general, are we thinking of the incoming signals, analysed for covariation under various heads such as motion, colour, orientation and so on, as fitting into the scheme as a whole?*]

The information needed for updating

Think, for example, of a human organization, say a sales organization. Out at the periphery there are any number of individual purchases being made; but the managing director, or his committee, don't want information about the individual purchases. They want information which will help them to make the high-order selections in the hierarchy of conditional policies for the organization. So, of course, only a tiny fraction of the informational traffic which impinges at the periphery of the organization reaches the high-level committee. My point is that if you had thought of the whole organization as an information *channel*, as those of us who started from communication engineering and communication theory might be tempted to do, you would find it derisorily inefficient. No doubt you could make something of a joke by pointing out how 'wasteful of information' is the

'channel' from the periphery to the managing director of the organization. But if you said it seriously and tried to persuade the managing
director that he ought to have a high capacity channel carrying all the
information from the periphery to his office, the joke would be on you.
For you would have missed the whole point of the organization.

In relation to the central nervous system, I think this is very important to keep in mind. Nothing is easier than to show that, viewed as an
information channel, the pathways from the retina to neurons deep in
the central nervous system carry only a fraction of the informational
traffic impinging on the sense receptors. As a joke we could describe
this as a 'terribly inefficient' system. But if we try to understand it as a
system whose function is to update the organization, then of course its
true efficiency would be measured by something quite inverse:
namely, the effectiveness with which it *prevents* information that is not
relevant to decision making from troubling the central system. Again,
you could make a joke of this and say that one of the main functions of
sensory information processing in the brain is to throw away information. But once we've smiled, let's see the point. That is what it is
designed to do. That is what it ought to do if it's to be biologically
effective. Measurement of information flow can be quite inept as a
guide to efficiency. If we keep this in mind it may throw a good deal of
light on the reasons for, and the probable functions of, the various
mechanisms.

In a hierarchic organization – and again to make this concrete keep
in mind the image of a human organization – how best can you
arrange to feed in information from the sensory systems to the different
levels of the organizing hierarchy? Through what kinds of processing
filters and computing operations should the information go with a view
to optimizing the state of readiness for action in the world in the
minimum time?

[*Let us consider in this light the two paths from the receptors to the
organizing system, that via FF and that via C in figure 3.2.*]

Processing the signals from the receptors

For the efficient planning of evaluated action, an agent needs information about the structured contents of his world, insofar as they set

constraints or enablements on the repertoire he means to use. How can the internal organizing process be most effectively guided by incoming stimuli? There are two extremes between which our solution can locate itself. The one extreme would be to install a bank of 'feature-filters' covering the whole range of possible inputs, so that each input became internally identifiable by the distribution of excitation, and appropriate logical networks could be installed to set up an appropriate state of readiness for each distribution. The other extreme would be to install a single self-adjusting 'imitator' of the input or some transform of the input, and allow it to fumble its way into balance with each input change under the guidance of a comparator or error indicator. Its setting would then determine the state of readiness. Suffice it here to say that whereas the first is wasteful of equipment unless all combinations of inputs are equally likely, the second is wasteful of time unless most combinations of inputs are highly unlikely. The best solution would seem to lie in a combination of the two principles, whereby 'feedforward' from relatively few key feature-filters is used to pre-select or mould the repertoire of the matching generator, on the basis of filtrates from both the incoming signals and the (multidimensional) error signals from the comparator.

As remarked earlier, the process of filtering and matching with comparison and error-feedback will of course be recognized as typical of much scientific investigation. Selected data suggest a hypothesis which generates a prediction; this prediction is then compared with data (usually including fresh material) and the discrepancies should ideally suggest refinements of the generative hypothesis.

If we agree that it is at least an open possibility that our own receptor systems are arranged in this way, then we will have to keep in mind two quite different possible sources of optical illusions and the various other informative psychophysical effects that we'll be looking at. On the one hand the sensory channel itself is likely to be plastic, being made of biological material. If you feed it with an abnormal sensory diet you may expect changes in its transfer characteristics which may give rise to perceptual illusions. An example of this is the familiar complementary after effect of looking at patches of different colours or the fact that after viewing a bright area a neutral test area looks locally dimmer.

On the other hand, figure 4.8 shows a familiar perceptual anomaly which I think it is fair to say is unlikely to be due to any anomalous

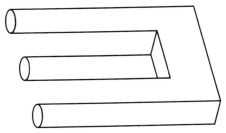

Figure 4.8   A well-known optical illusion which seems likely to reflect a mismatch on the 'response' side of the brain.

process at the retina or in the input side. Here one could say that the author has wickedly drawn the thing so that the internal mechanism for matching your readiness to the object gets conflicting clues; and in terms of the concept of perception I have been advocating, one would look on the response side of the organization of your brain, rather than on the input side, for the physiological correlates of the subjective anomaly: two incompatible subroutines are finding themselves invoked.

So what I am suggesting is that we should think of the modelling of perception not in terms of an exclusive choice between filtering and internal adaptive matching by the internal replication of the input, but in terms of an interaction of both. Many observed effects seem to indicate that perception is indeed a synthetic activity, one guided by cues extracted by the filter mechanisms; but what we see has many elements which come from the structure within rather than from the stimulus without. [*What part, then, do the signals from the sense organs play in our perceptions?*]

Pitfalls of perceptual psychophysiology

I open my eyes, my occipital cortex is stimulated, I see a world of objects. How can we connect these facts? Is it proper to say, for example, that I am 'really' witnessing my brain activity? Is perceiving some kind of internal *observation* of incoming signals from our sense organs? It was for some time thought obvious that this was the case. In the classic case of colour vision, for example, the correspondence between the psychophysical data and photometric curves for the sensory receptors is dramatically close.[3]

When the physical intensity of a sound is increased, it is perceived as 'louder'. What should the physiologist expect to find happening in the brain as the correlate of this experience? We may expect that *some* change must occur in the firing pattern of some neural activity, but there are a bewildering variety of candidate codes to be considered. The frequency in some fibres, or the number of fibres that are active, may increase with perceived loudness; they could equally well decrease (Segundo, 1970). The effect of increased intensity might be only to increase the regularity or coherence of firing while leaving the mean frequency unchanged; and so on. It may be plausible to expect the perception of an increase in intensity to correlate with some over-all measure of neural activity, but it is far from necessary.

With some relief, we learn from physiology that in *peripheral* sensory neurons the overall firing rate does increase with intensity. Can we, then, treat the subjective data as a kind of internal measurement of this firing rate? If so, we might expect the loudness that is psychophysically estimated to vary with physical intensity according to the same law as the average neural firing rate.

If one asks a subject to estimate the loudness of a sound or the brightness of a light, or the stiffness of a trigger, by putting a number to it, most subjects choose numbers related to the physical intensity according to a power law. This is 'Stevens's law' and holds across many modalities (Stevens, 1957, 1961).

It has been known for a long time, however, that in general the physiological response of a sense organ is not power law related, but roughly logarithmically related to the intensity of the stimulus, I, so that the firing frequency,

$$f = k \log I$$

over a certain range. What is more, if one derives a scale of 'subjective intensity' as Fechner (1862) did, by assuming that just noticeable differences (JNDs) are subjectively equal, then since most JNDs are proportional to physical intensity the resulting scale is logarithmic. On the presupposition that perception is the witnessing of incoming impulses, it was perhaps natural to take Fechner's law as a corroboration of the physiological law. Accordingly, when Stevens produced his power law, both he and his opponents tended to interpret it as throwing doubt on the logarithmic law of receptor response.

If one drops the idea that perception is the witnessing of incoming signals, the problem loosens up. As suggested above, we look for the correlate of psychophysical properties not in the incoming stream or its derivatives but in the matching changes elicited in the organizing system. On this view, when a subject estimates sensory intensity, the neural correlate of his perceptual experience would be an internally generated matching response, automatically adjusted so that (in at least some respects) its internal effects are equal and opposite to the internal disturbance produced by the sensory input.

The perceived intensity of the stimulus might plausibly be related to the physical intensity of the internal effort required to generate the matching response, rather than to the sensory input itself. Suppose, for example, that the matching response generator had a logarithmic characteristic like that of the sensory transducer, so that its output

$$f_m = k_m \log \Psi$$

where Ψ represents the internal effort; and that the sensory transducer output $f_s = k_s \log I$. Then assuming that in the psychophysical tasks devised by Stevens, f_m is adjusted by the supervisory system to equal f_s, we will have $k_m \log \Psi = k_s \log I$, or $\Psi \propto I^\beta$, where $\beta = k_s/k_m$. Thus if we adopt a matching response model, logarithmic transfer characteristics can easily lead to a power law relationship between stimulus intensity I and the internal 'supervisory effort'.

It is too early to say whether this is what goes on in the information system of a subject estimating intensities of stimulation; but at least it shows how one and the same model could account for both Stevens's power law and the logarithmic functions of Fechner and the physiologists. It also shows how arbitrary it would be in general to equate perceived intensity with firing rate of sensory inflow.

We must beware of regarding all the subjective phenomena that we meet as some sort of privileged way of witnessing the phsyiological events in our retinae [*(and other sense organs)*]. Optical illusions may have their origin at many levels in the information processing system. The old question – is what we see 'really' on the retina or 'really' in the external world? – is a philosophical howler: a badly posed question. Seeing, I have been suggesting, is matching one's state of organization to the visually mediated demands of the world. The only location for what is seen is in that world. (Even when a visual experience is artificially induced by electrical brain stimulation, the *perceived* location of what is seen is out in front of the subject.) Your retina is one of the links in the chain of demand on your brain organization; and the *physical correlates* of what you see have, of course, their locations all along that chain. But I can't imagine any circumstances in which it would make sense to say that *what we see* is located 'at' the retina, rather than 'at' the visual cortex, or halfway down the light path from our eyes to the object. Forgive me for having laboured what may seem obvious, but it is sometimes neglected in psychophysiological discussions with confusing results.

Perception is more than classificatory behaviour

[*This final section was addressed to designers of artefacts capable of pattern 'recognition' and so approaches the concerns of this chapter from another angle.*]

The kinship of interest between the designers of automata and theorists of perception has led to a remarkably fruitful series of interactions; but there are subtle differences of emphasis between the two sides which have also, I think, tended towards a confounding of a distinction. I mean the distinction between perception as experience and perception as behaviour, as the manifestation of input-output coordination. To see that this distinction is one of fact and not merely of linguistic convention, it is only necessary to remind ourselves of all the bodily processes which come into the category of input-output coordination (we have mentioned already the matching of pupil diameter to the intensity of light) yet are unaccompanied by conscious perception. Similarly there are many processes of an artificial kind which are discriminatory, classificatory, and so on, where it would seem a little perverse to speak of perception. A sieve, for example, will receive an input and will nicely classify it into categories according to size, but few of us would regard it as *perceiving* what it handles. Throughout the world there are in fact any number of more complex natural processes which can be regarded as classificatory, but it would be very odd indeed to call them perceptual. For example, wherever water dribbles from the end of a drain pipe or the edge of a rock and the wind is blowing, the heavier drops are deflected a short distance, and the smaller drops a greater distance. So here is 'classification' going on – but who would be so animistic as to call it an instance of perception?

What I am suggesting, then, is that in our models the mere

appearance of internal configurations which match or correspond one for one to features of the environment, though it may be a necessary feature of any model of perception, does not *ipso facto* guarantee that perceiving is going on in these models, nor that what is going on is in any sense an adequate model of what goes on in people's nervous systems when they perceive.

A percept can be thought of as a current *constraint on the organization of action* by the perceiver. What I perceive becomes a datum for my calculation of any action or reaction to which its presence is relevant. The observable evidence of my having perceived it is usually, therefore, the correlation observed in my behaviour between output and input, provided that I am suitably motivated to show this. (Anyone who experiments on perception knows that the real problem is to make sure that the subject is, in fact, motivated to show the coordination in which we are interested.)

Typical perceptual tasks are those of discrimination, classification, matching; and in each case the study is conducted trying to ensure that the subject is motivated to perform an action whose form will reflect the feature which we want him to perceive. Because such input–output correlations are often required in industry for practical purposes, there is then a temptation to take any device which shows the appropriate correlation between input and output as *ipso facto* a possible explanatory model of perceptual processes in a living organism, so reducing the problem of perception to a problem of discriminative, classificatory public behaviour, leaving out the awkward questions of motivation to action and the experience of the perceiving agent. I want to suggest that as the study of perception advances we will need to sharpen this distinction between perception and mere 'input–output coordination'. . . .

If we are interested in artefacts

The point I would stress in summary is that in most of our artefacts the work of conscious, normative behaviour is intended to be performed by someone else. Normally we design our automata to subserve ultimate goals which are not autonomously determined: they are set by ourselves. Most of our automata need not, and normally should not, have any autonomous supervisory system, so they lack an essential feature of conscious agency. Hence the suggestion that not all features of models of human perception which try to do justice to the *experienced* aspects of it are necessarily relevant to the design of artefacts required to develop sensori-motor coordination. Conversely there is no guarantee that the most effective solution of this design problem may have any claim on the attention of psychologists. In other words, oddly enough, automaton designers with an interest in perception of speech and visual form might do well to ignore, in the first instance, those aspects of the psychological theory of perception that are primarily concerned with perceiving; for perceiving is something that their automata may not be required to do.

If, on the other hand, we are interested in perception

We must take into account not only the physical correlate of *classification*, but also the correlate of *action*, and the part played by the percept in the planning of action. All of these have to make their appearance in our model before we could even begin to advance it as a candidate for the explanation of perception.

Finally, we should beware of assuming too readily that the 'feature-filters' we find in the nervous system are acting as classifiers of input patterns. They may have to do with quite other functions, such as the control of eye movements and accommodation; and even when they supply the perceptual system their job may only be to initiate and guide the exploratory matching activity whose successful achievement is the act of recognition.

Notes

1 For discussion of the points of difference between ocular and tactile exploration, especially as regards the saccadic hops made by the eyes (as opposed to smooth stroking), see MacKay (1973b).
2 On this view the otherwise puzzling 'bluntness' of tuning of many cortical units acquires a natural explanation: for maximal informational efficiency an associative net whose task is to look out for what covaries with what 'should receive inputs extracted by filters sufficiently broadly tuned to optimise their information rate' (MacKay 1985b).
3 There are counter-examples. D. Regan (1968) has found that when a subject views an unpatterned flickering field, the corresponding brain waves are present well above the frequency at which flicker ceases to be perceptible.

5

Seeing is not Believing

Perceptual anomalies as clues to brain function

Let us move to the practical question: how can we systematically learn some things about brain organization from the study of our visual perceptual experience? Here let me just say that visual experience, like the rest of our experience, is most instructive when something goes wrong with it. That is true about even a TV set. As long as you look at a well-functioning TV picture, you learn very little about how the TV system works, but if you see the frame start drifting up, as it sometimes does, you begin to realize that you are dealing with a synchronous system and you can work out the frequency of synchronization and so on. It is in this spirit that we look for illusions and disorders of perception as clues to what kind of processing machinery is at work. Our first demonstration was known to the Greeks.

Optical speedometers: the 'waterfall' after-effect

On a very slowly rotating gramophone turntable we have a circle of paper spotted with large ink blobs. If you watch the centre for about 20 to 30 seconds, what you are doing is allowing parts of your retina to be optically 'stroked' by images moving always in the same direction in any given location. Now if your visual system contains 'speedometers', little computing networks which are sensitive to the velocity of the optical image in each region of the retina, then it would not be surprising if giving them a prolonged diet of one particular direction of motion would result in a kind of backlash effect, such that when you provide a neutral input you see the negative of the velocity that you previously saw. When you have been looking at it long enough test this out by looking away at some other object – the wall or somebody's face – and with luck you should see the area that was occupied by the rotating disk rotating backwards.

You notice that although there is apparent motion, there is no displacement. Although every point in the field previously stimulated by the moving surface seems to be moving, one is simultaneously aware that its position is unchanged. In terms of an 'internal image' of the world, of course, this makes no sense. No unitary physical display could exhibit this dissociation between velocity and change of position, familiar though it is as a formal device in physics. Once we drop the idea of a 'screen of consciousness', however, and think of perception as the internal updating of the organizing system to match filtrates of the incoming stimuli, the problem assumes a more tractable form. Relieved of the need to re-integrate all optical information in a unitary display, we can readily envisage how different features of an optical image (such as motion, position, colour, orientation) might be filtered off to evoke or modify adaptive responses in quite different circuits of the integrated organizing system. It then becomes easy to see how abnormal adaptation of the subsystem handling one such feature, such as motion, might give rise to mutually conflicting perceptions (incompatible adjustments of different circuits of the organizing system).

Central and peripheral vision differ radically

Here is another demonstration which makes rather a different point although the stimulus is much the same. We use the turntable again and a pattern of large black blobs or a ray pattern as in figure 5.1. Stare steadily, not this time at the centre, but at a point in the room some 10 to 20 degrees away, and observe what happens while the gramophone turns; what you'll find is that over the next 5 to 15 seconds the rotating picture slows down. You see it as going slower and slower and eventually (after some 15 seconds) the ray figure will begin to disintegrate; the rays will begin to crumple like a flag waving in the wind. And yet, if you move your eyes from the position you have been staring at to any other position in the room (even near to your original fixation spot) you will find that the disk flips back into normal motion.

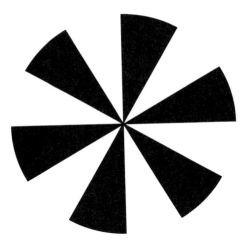

Figure 5.1   Ray figure with broad sectors.

The interesting thing is that if you do as you were doing in the earlier demonstration and use a part of the retina near your point of fixation as the area on which the rotating image falls, you find no such fragmentation. So what we have got here is evidence that the computing networks that are attached to the periphery of the visual field (i.e. from about $2\frac{1}{2}$ degrees off-centre outwards) have quite a different dynamics – they work on different principles from those connected to the centre of the visual field.

Now these are not terribly exciting points but they illustrate the methodology. What we are doing is looking for anomalies, illusions, oddities, malfunctionings of perception which can give us clues to the questions we ought to ask as physiologists. We don't stop where I have just stopped: we immediately go into the lab or ask someone at the lab, 'can you see signs that, when you look at the peripheral connected system, it has different dynamics of the sort that you would expect from this subjective experience?' So there is a to-and-fro traffic between the experimental psychology of visual perception, which has studied things like this for years, and the neurophysiology of the information processing of the visual system.

Electrical stimulation of cortex

Plate 16 relates to a rather dramatic illustration of this two-way traffic. The anomaly is here produced by imposing electrical activity on the organization within the brain. The X-ray photograph is of the skull of a blind nurse who is hale and well. She volunteered to allow the neurosurgeons and physiologists Brindley and Lewin to implant 80 little radio receivers under her scalp and to run an 80-way cable to 80 little electrodes over the visual part of her brain right at the back of the head on the right side.

What they then did was selectively to stimulate one receiver at a time and ask her what she saw. Sure enough she did 'see': she was able when one receiver was stimulated, as she sat in front of an audience, to point and say 'I see a spot of light up there'; and when another was stimulated unknown to her, she said 'Oh, it's like a grain of rice over there' (pointing to a different position). So there was a very direct relation between the position of certain restricted physical interference with her visual system and her conscious experience. On the other hand, combinations of signals (such as three dots in a triangle) very often produced bizarre and unintelligible effects rather than the sort of patterns that might have turned out to be an aid to her in her blindness. Nevertheless, the experiment did give rise to a lot of evidence of a new sort, and is a pointer which is being followed up still. For example, when the lady was asked, 'move your eyes and tell me whether the spot of light moves or not', she was able to say, 'yes it moves; it was over there; it is now over there'. When she moved her eyes to the left the spot of light seemed to move to the left – a nice bit of extra evidence in the general discussion (see preceding chapter) of how the visual world stays stable and the basis on which we perceive movement.

Two demonstrations using a detuned TV receiver

There is a third sort of phenomenon. Here the reorganization is imposed to some extent by the perceiving subject, in a rather curious way.

Switch your television receiver to an empty channel so that you have on the screen a random speckle, a formless twinkling snowstorm.

1 If you lay on the screen a transparency of a highly repetitive pattern like the ray figure (figure 4.3), you see a rotating rosette and if you *think* about it you can change the direction of rotation. [*(Alternatively view the twinkling screen by reflection in a sheet of clear glass held at an angle to the TV screen and set figure 4.3 a few inches behind the glass.)*] So here we have got organization imposed in some sense by *you*. What

we are doing now is imposing a certain state of organization – a state of strain you might say, certainly a state of cooperativity – on your visual network by imposing the regularity of this particular pattern on the screen.

2 Here is a second demonstration using the random snowstorm. Take a circle of wire or a slim ring of black card about 6 inches in diameter, hold it against the TV screen and move it around. The snowstorm of boiling noise becomes 'attached' to the card and moves around the screen with it. If now you place your finger on the screen within the ring of card and continue moving the card do you see how your finger has locked the noise to it, where previously it was moving?

Again what we have got here is imposed structure. But structure imposed on what? Not on what is happening on the screen, of course! That would be superstition. The activity on the screen remains entirely random: nothing changes there when we bring up figure 4.3 or the black ring. What we are imposing is a structure on *your* conditional readiness to reckon with what is on the screen. The imposition is the result of activity in your own brain.

One reason for looking at this, and it is a point we shall come back to, is to show why I insisted in the first chapter that we should be careful about not breaking up hyphens. Because if I were to ask you, 'where is this happening that you have just seen; where is the movement going on that clings to the circle of card?', I put it to you that you would have to say it is on the screen. There is nowhere else for it to be. So the question, 'where is the movement-perceived?' (hyphenated), is answered by saying, 'on the screen'. While the question, 'where is the physical-correlate-of-the-changes-in-your-conscious-experience when I do this?', is answered, 'well, obviously, inside your head'. It would be bizarre to suppose it is anywhere else, although nobody has looked for it.

What we are saying is that there is an important operational difference between talking about the 'where' of perceiving and the 'where' of correlated information processing activity: in the first case the subject is I, the perceiver, and we are talking essentially I-story language; in the second case the subject is the brain and the locus is the brain. You remember my science-fiction example of the brain in the wheelbarrow that is wheeled out into the garden – you see now that this kind of experience with the snowstorm makes the same point in a different way.

The McCollough effect

You have probably looked, from time to time, at the front cover of this book, so you may already notice faint pink or green colouration on various areas of figure 5.2. If you run your eyes around the front cover for about 10 minutes (keeping the book always the same way up) you will probably find that you see a somewhat stronger after-effect; your visual system generates an imposed state of re-adaptation such that the upper triangle of figure 5.2 looks pinkish and the lower greenish. Moreover, you will find that the after-effect lasts for several hours (rather than the seconds that one is accustomed to in the case of most other visual and auditory after-effects).

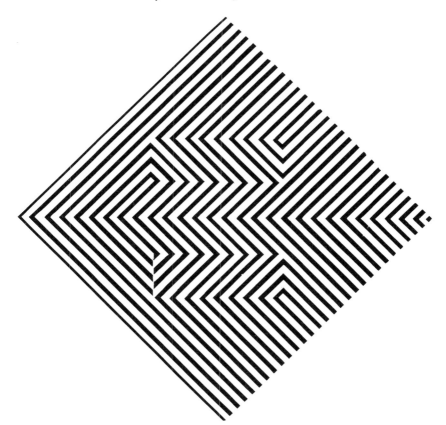

Figure 5.2   A McCollough test figure.

This is the McCollough effect, discovered less than 30 years ago. It is a very exciting demonstration that not just central neural tissue of the sort that we would expect to be associated with memory can adapt to steady conditions of this kind, but even uni-ocular visual tissue. If you had used only one eye and exposed it to the red and green patterns then you would have seen the colour difference with that eye but not with the other eye. So even the peripheral nervous system attached to one of the two eyes can adapt in this way. I might have called it 'learning' but learning would not be the right word because what is actually learned is the opposite of what was previously seen. Where you previously saw '2 o'clock' orientation as really looking green you now, as the after-effect, see '2 o'clock' as looking pinkish. So it is a negative learning, if you like.

My wife and I some years ago discovered that if, immediately after a 15 minute exposure to the coloured stripes, you cover the eye with a black patch and 24 hours later take the patch off, the after-effect is still at full strength. So this is not just a matter of transient physiological fatigue in cells that are sensitive to both colour and orientation. This is a genuine change in the synaptic strength or something in the visual hook-up attached to that one eye, such that unless you feed other information in that overwrites it, the synaptic hook-up is semi-permanent (at least on the scale of 24 hours). So here you have a model of the physiology of learning in the peripheral visual system.

What is common to all these things is that unless we were prepared to talk psychology – to ask people about conscious experience – we, as *physiologists*, would not know anything about them. There was a time, you see, when scientists were, as they thought, purists in ruling conscious experience out from science. Psychology had to pretend to be like physics in order to be respectable. That fashion, I hope, is gone for ever, because it is so obvious now how much faster you can get on in understanding things like the visual system if you are prepared to study conscious experience and take the hints that optical illusions and other things give you, as well as the physiology.

Three examples of internally generated reorganization

We have so far been looking at imposed or acquired reorganization. Let us proceed to three examples of internally generated organization – or reorganization.

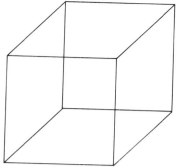

Figure 5.3   Necker cube.

Necker cube   The first is a simple line drawing of a box, known as the Necker cube because the German psychologist L. A. Necker first drew attention to its interesting behaviour.

You can perceive it as a box with the lowest horizontal line forming the lower edge of the vertical face of the cube which is closest to you (the cube is then slightly below the line of sight). But even as you are thinking about this, the cube is likely to flip so that the same line becomes the lower edge of the *rear* panel of the cube (the cube then seeming to be viewed from slightly below). If you fixate the middle of the cube you will see it flipping from one mode to the other. What you have are two *conditional readinesses to reckon with it* which are equally good matches to the incoming data. I put it to you that what you are seeing as it flips is the conscious experience which is the correlate of the presence of two subroutines in the organizing system. The supervisory system is bringing these subroutines up to match the demands set by the lines on the page and each subroutine matches equally well, so, having had its go, it flops back and the other one comes up.

If you take a piece of card and use it as a shutter to cut off your view of figure 5.3 in a regular manner, you will find that you can settle to a rate (around one to two interruptions per second) at which you can voluntarily make the cube flip from looking one way to looking the other in time with the uncovering of the picture.

Here again your thinking about it is efficacious in bringing about a change in your conditional readiness. And when I say conditional readiness you realize just what the word 'conditional' now means: you are not in fact going to do anything about it, I guarantee, but *if* you had to make a model – say a 3-D matchstick model – of what you see you are ready to do it with the thing placed slightly below *or* above the line of sight. So this is another example of the way in which subjective experience of perception can reveal activities which doubtless have their correlates in brain function.

Embossed Maltese cross   In plate 15 we are perceiving – in the sense of 'setting up a conditional readiness to reckon with' – something that is normally lit. And 'normally lit' here evidently means lit from above. [*(Turn the book upside down to see which sculpture is sticking out and which is indented.)*]

This is an illustration of the high degree of convergence or cooperativity in your nervous system between different sorts of analyser of the visual input. In this case it must be a rather abstract, but biologically very important, analyser of where the light is coming from or what a shadow means, which cooperates with the geometrical cues to give us this oddly biased experience.

Dalmatian dog   Some of you may immediately see figure 5.4 as a Dalmatian dog on a snowy or leafy pavement, others may not, for it sometimes takes a while, if you have not seen it before, to see it. The dog, seen from his left side, fills most of the middle of the picture: his muzzle is to the ground and a black ear dangling. The point is, you have to have a certain, we might say, 'perceptual readiness' to perceive it. There are other patterns which are more difficult than this to make sense of, in terms of a conditional readiness to reckon with an object. People can get angry with each other over the obviousness that some of them claim for them, while others 'see and see and never perceive', if I may use a biblical expression. I think the same point applies, by the way (and we will come back to it), that having the facts in front of you is not a sufficient condition for perceiving, because perceiving is not at all a matter of itemizing the facts.

Perceiving . . .

Perceiving is a matter of generating a matching response. We have seen with the Necker cube how in even that crude situation we may

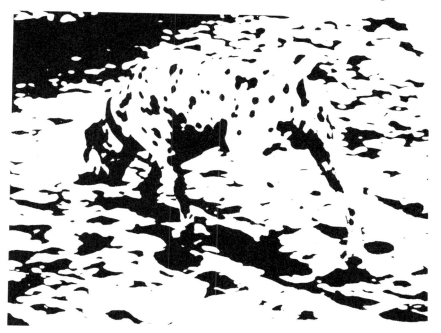

Figure 5.4   Dalmatian dog. Photo by R. C. James.

have two matching responses that are equally good. In a case like the Dalmatian dog some folk may never – if they are sufficiently ill-equipped – hit on the appropriate matching response to produce the conditional readiness to reckon with the object, which, once you have observed it, is quite verifiably present in the scene that is making the demands on your state of conditional readiness.

. . . And wishful perceiving

Notice the distinction between this and wishful thinking. There are such things as Rorschach blot tests where you put tea leaves or other abstract patterns in front of somebody and force them to tell you what it reminds them of. Here wishful thinking or arbitrary and baseless perceptual enterprises are very much a matter of the individual subject and there is nothing very inter-subjective in the result. In the case of the Dalmatian dog, however, the situation is perfectly inter-subjective: you could find the original photo – in fact find the original dog – and have to agree that, if you failed to see it, that was your fault because it really was there. So when we talk about wishful thinking we are talking about something more than the readiness to generate. Readiness to generate the matching response is a necessary condition of perceiving but it is not a sufficient condition. Wishful thinking is a readiness to generate a matching response in the absence of adequate demand. (The 'adequate demand' may not be sensory demand; more of that later.)

Believing and perceiving

It is time to ask ourselves: if seeing is not believing then what is believing? Or rather, where does a concept like believing come in terms of our skeleton information-flow map? I think it is fairly obvious that insofar as belief, in general, shapes conditional readiness, the organizing system must implicitly represent the agent's beliefs (although of course the supervisory system which operates at a higher level of abstraction will also represent many of the agent's beliefs).

You may ask: then what is the difference between believing and perceiving? The difference is that the updating activity in perceiving is in matching response to feedforward from the sensory input (tactile, visual or whatever). It is because the supervisory system tests for match and gets an 'OK' that this state of conditional readiness is dynamically linked to the scanning readinesses of the eye and so forth and is hallmarked with vision, touch or whatever.

Beliefs are represented implicitly by the conditional readinesses that result from, and are left over after, the episode of updating. So when you look around the room and see someone is there and then shut your eyes, you still *believe* he is there because your conditional readiness to reckon with his being there has not yet evaporated but you are no longer matching a sensory demand in maintaining it. So the embodiment of our beliefs, I am suggesting, is the state of conditional readiness to reckon with the world after the updating process in matching response to sensory demands (or apart from that updating process).

There will be a need to go into this matter of the embodiment of beliefs in much more detail later.

The costs of knowing

What I am suggesting has, of course, one very interesting consequence with which I want to conclude this chapter. It is that knowing, believing and so on have physical costs. There is, on this view, no knowing, no believing, no learning – or unlearning even – without a physical change in the structure which embodies your state of conditional readiness to reckon with the world, because it is in and through changes of your state of conditional readiness to reckon with the world that all experienced changes in your beliefs are embodied. Our assumption – the brain scientist's working assumption of chapter 1 – entails the fact that knowing and believing have physical costs.

Let us think about the logical consequence of this. Suppose a super-scientist were able to look into your brain, so as to establish, with the aid of instruments, in every detail your current state of conditional readiness which embodies all that you know and believe to be the case. This is science fiction, but let us suppose that he can do this with a videotape and camera and everything else so that later on he can bring it round and show it to you and verify that this was an up to date and scientific job. Note that what we are discussing at the moment is not at all whether the super-scientist can predict to you what you will believe. What we are discussing – with the eye of a logician – is the cognitive status, or if you like, the logical claim to your assent, of what he ultimately decides to put down as an accurate representation of the case at the present moment.

So we make the science-fiction assumption that the super-scientist has now an accurate and complete depiction of the state of your conditional readiness. Question: would *you* be correct to believe it? Well, you say, why not, if he has done his job properly? But think – there is a physical cost to any change in what you *believe*: our working assumption is that no change can take place in what you believe without a correlated change in your state of conditional readiness. If then his representation of your state of conditional readiness is accurate *now* it will necessarily be inaccurate if *you* believe it. Like Tristram Shandy's attempt to write a diary of writing a diary of his life, it is a nonsense for you to wish you knew the up to date condition of your state of conditional readiness. There is no such story that you would be correct to believe (except of course in retrospect as relating to a past time). Furthermore, if our super-scientist in this science-fiction world were able to make a predictive model (and there is no reason in principle why he should not), which covered not only the present moment but the next few seconds or minutes, *he* might be correct to believe that prediction, but you would be mistaken to believe it if you knew it.

Logical relativity

What I am sketching – and we shall hear more of this – is the bare bones of a principle of relativity. It is like the physical principle of relativity which we all know about in general terms, which says that if one physical observer, travelling at a particular speed, is to be correct in what he says about a particular situation, he must *not* believe and say the same as another observer moving with a different velocity in relation to that situation. In order that each should be correct, what they believe must be different.

Oddly enough, out of nothing more than the working assumption whose consequences we are exploring, an analogous principle of logical relativity applies to the current and immediately future states of any conscious cognitive agent's state of conditional readiness. *No completely up to date or predictive specification of that agent's state of conditional readiness exists unknown to him, which has for him an unconditional claim to assent, i.e. such that if only he knew it he would be correct.* On the contrary, any completely accurate specification of your state of conditional readiness has, if I may coin a term, a 'disclaim' to your assent. It is not merely that it hasn't got a claim, it actively disclaims your assent. The same basis on which it can be verified to be correct for outside observers is the basis on which it can be verified that *you* would be mistaken to believe it. It is something that you would be mistaken to believe, because your believing it would make it false.

As a consequence, then, of our embodiment in the physical world, knowing and believing have physical costs. The physical costs of knowing are such as to render indeterminate for A, the agent, the view that O predictively takes. This is a tough one. It goes against all our intuition – as with physical relativity theory. We all know the outrage that was caused when Einstein suggested that what one observer, moving at a certain speed relative to a massive particle, was correct to believe about its mass, could not be and must not be the same as what another observer moving with a different velocity would be correct to believe about it. People said 'nonsense, you are just contradicting yourself', because everybody had grown up with a Newtonian absolute space–time frame in which everything had one and only one true description. I hope that physics has now gone through that phase and is content to recognize that relativity does not mean self-contradiction, provided you label for standpoint the beliefs that are correct.

What I am saying is that, in the case of persons and their actions, you must label for standpoint the proposition whose validity you want to assess, before you can say whether it is valid or not. The standpoint of the observer is logically different from the standpoint of the agent – so radically that what O would be correct to believe is what A would be mistaken to believe. In that, there is a direct parallel with physical relativity: both are counter-intuitive but, I think, both are inescapable. So we are in a very odd situation indeed, logically, in trying to make models of ourselves. As we go on in subsequent chapters we shall see that this point has consequences which will be more and more interesting and certainly not insignificant.

Concepts of 'truth'

Another way of putting it is this: we really have to face an ambiguity in the concept of truth with which we all grew up. We all grew up with the idea, formally or otherwise expressed, that if anyone is correct in believing a proposition P, everyone would be correct in believing it. P can be labelled unambiguously 'true' or 'false': logicians use 'T' and 'F', or '1' and '0'. I am perfectly happy to do this in the whole wide world of propositions about reality and imagined reality *except* propositions about cognitive agents' cognitive states. The cognitive agent's cognitive state *cannot* – logically – have one unique label 'true' or 'false' such that from its being called 'true' you can conclude that anyone and everyone would be correct to believe it.

Now that gives us an option in logic. One way is to take the boot-faced logician's approach and say P is true if it corresponds with the situation it describes. Now that sounds perfectly fair, doesn't it? I would suggest that we keep the word *accurate* for that and say: P is accurate if it corresponds to the situation it describes. Because there is another use of the word true which is operationally, I suspect, much more important, and certainly one I would want to preserve at all costs: namely, that P is *true* only if anyone and everyone would be correct to *believe* it. If P is such that you would be incorrect to believe it, P is *untruthful*. That is perhaps a good adjective to bring out. If the boot-faced logician insists that he likes his 'T' to stand for true, I don't mind as long as he calls it 'true$_1$' or the like, but he has then to accept that 'true$_1$' propositions can be untruthful. Well, OK, so be it. I'm suggesting that we go easy on the word truth, that we use it only when we are safe, and that we talk on the one hand about the *accuracy* of a description of your cognitive system and on the other about its *belief-worthiness* or otherwise. This use of terms will allow us to explore the possibility that an account of your state of conditional readiness may be accurate on the one hand but also unbeliefworthy for you.

This, you see, is where it becomes useful to recognize what I have called a principle of relativity such that when the observer, the super-scientist, is correct to believe what *he* believes about your state of conditional readiness, we can then ask, what is it that *you* would be correct to believe about it? Because you certainly would not be correct to believe *his* story. And the answer, as I am going to be arguing later, is that you would be correct to believe that the immediate future of your state of conditional readiness, in part, is *up to you* to determine.

6

Reading the Mind

So far we have looked mainly at the interface between the external world and the organism. We have looked at the sense organs and the way in which the information from them is processed. We have considered some of the kinds of conscious experiences we have as a result and the kind of light that our conscious experiences can throw on the machinery that mediates this mysterious process. We have been looking at the ways in which the external world can find itself internally represented in the information-flow system of the organism. But, of course, human beings, and I daresay other animals too, are not just stimulus driven. We have an ongoing mental life even in the absence of, or regardless of, external stimuli, and so as we study the brain we want to ask ourselves whether we can next track down the physical correlates of this ongoing, covert, mental life.

Mental activities: a topographical arrangement within the brain?

Phrenology is regarded nowadays as outdated. It was supposed to be a scientific way of determining where mental activity went on, by looking for bumps on the surface of the head. We don't take it seriously now, but on the other hand it is a very reasonable question whether the correlates of various mental activities – which we imagine are there to be studied if only we knew how to – are localized or not. When we conduct mental activities such as thinking, imagining things, working out problems, are the correlates in our brains smeared out, so to speak, over the whole thing, so that we have to wave our hands and use the magic word 'holistic' and say that the brain 'as a whole' conducts the correlated operations? Or can we find something more topographically organized as the correlates of mental activity, as we did when we were thinking about seeing and hearing and other things that are stimulus driven?

In chapter 3 we built up a minimal information-flow map for self-organization and you might well ask whether we can use this as a pointer to the way more complex mental activity might be distributed. The flow map, as I pointed out earlier, looks very like the sort of diagram you might draw to indicate how nerve fibres run from one point to another in the brain, but we mustn't assume there will be any direct correspondence of that sort. There used to be a form of gas thermostat which consisted simply of an expanding sphere, a balloon, sitting in a part of the gas supply pipe which was warmed by the gas burner. The lines of cause and effect drawn by the information engineer in that case would not correspond to any pipes or connections in the gas thermostat. Similarly here, although we might be lucky and find that there were geographically isolated regions we could identify, it is not something that we can take for granted.

Locating experimentally the 'seat' of covert mental activities

To get further data then, on this question of whether there is any localization of brain function in covert mental activity, we have to go back to experiment. Here the classic work of Wilder Penfield is one of the best pointers to what can be hoped for. Penfield was operating to relieve epilepsy and before destroying any defective tissue he wanted to know where he was *functionally* in the brain. The patient's head was open, the skull partially reflected back under local anaesthetic. The patient was conscious and able to report the effects of having electric current fed into one part of the brain or another. Penfield stimulated, for example, at the back of the head (see plate 3) with 60 cycle electric current, and the patient reported visual sensations. Stimulation in Broca's area on the left not far from the ear lobe, or further back in Wernicke's area, could result in the blockage of the capacity to speak.

But most dramatically, when he stimulated in parts of the temporal lobe in many of these patients, the patients, while not losing their awareness that they were in the operating theatre in Montreal, would bear witness to experiencing past events. One, for example, felt she was back home in the tenement building, hearing the kids calling at the foot of the stairs. Another reported being back on the farm in South Africa talking with friends. This replay, as it were, of earlier experience resulted from stimulation in the temporal area but not in other areas.

So one way in which we can do some crude mapping is to feed current into the system and find out what mental activities are either induced or blocked as a result. This allows us to get a vague impression of localization. But of course the method is drastic – you have to have the skull open – and the question we come back to is whether there are less drastic ways of making the skull 'transparent'.

Nuclear magnetic resonance imaging (MRI)

Plate 17 shows an early picture using a currently valuable clinical method. Using the nuclear magnetic resonance principle (which physics developed for other purposes) you can study the layout of the brain in a conscious individual without invading his system at all. Scanning from various directions, and using a computer to work out the strength of the resonances in the molecules through which the testing beam is passing, different parts of the brain show up as having slightly differing chemical constitutions. With this method, as you can see, you can get a very good indication of the gross geography inside the head. So the head is made transparent in that sense, but this method does not of itself allow you to monitor the *activity* that is going on.[1]

PET scanning

By using positron emission tomography (PET) scanning, one can derive functional maps showing how the activity is distributed during various mental operations. Oxygen containing a short-lived radioactive isotope is injected into the bloodstream of the subject. Within the following 2 minutes most of the radioactive atoms disintegrate, each emitting two positrons in opposite directions. A ring of coincidence counters around the subject's head allows a back-computation to be made of the position of each atom when it disintegrated.

Plate 18 (from a colleague at the Hammersmith MRC Cyclotron unit in London) shows four levels of the active brain while the subject is lying quietly. In black are shown (top row) the cerebral blood flow and (bottom row) the oxygen uptake. There is a pretty close correspondence; evidently the blood flow is kept matched to the demands of the tissues. You can see how the regions which are rich in neurons take up much more oxygen than the white matter in each 'slice'.

Using this positron emission tomography method while the subject engaged in various mental tasks, Phelps, Mazziotta and colleagues at the University of California in Los Angeles have been able to see well-localized concentrations of activity needing energy in different areas during the different tasks. In plate 19 (see also the back cover of this book) the arrowed areas are those where the highest rate of oxygen uptake is occurring. The five ways in which the subject's mind was occupied were as follows:

1 *Visual*.   The subject was looking at visual stimuli. The occipital area at the back of the head shows the highest level of uptake (red).
2 *Auditory*.   In response to auditory input Herschel's gyrae light up.
3 *Cognitive*.   With the subject solving a complex mental problem, the frontal regions of the brain light up indicating that cells there were working abnormally hard and consuming more oxygen.
4 *Memory*.   The subject was read a story, having been told that he would be rewarded if he could repeat the story accurately afterwards. For this memory task there are indications that the hippocampus, one of the lower structures of the brain, was especially active. (This picture is of a lower slice of the brain than the others.)
5 *Motor*.   Then there was a motor task: alternate finger/thumb movements with the right hand. This activated the primary sensory motor cortex.

In this way, at least over a short time (the isotope that is used does not last many minutes), you can accumulate evidence that certain parts of the brain really are more concerned in certain forms of mental activity than others.

Electro-encephalography (EEG)

The electrical method, familiar from hospital EEG, provides an alternative to the above two methods. [*Perhaps one should say a complementary technique, rather than an alternative, for while MRI and PET scans can offer location in all three dimensions within the head, EEG currently offers time resolution which is superior by two orders of magnitude.*]

The problem, however, for electrical brain recording has always been that the brain has a great deal of activity going on which is easy to record but which has very little to do with local processing of information in the sense that we are talking about. So the response to most stimuli is embedded in a constant buzz of unrelated activity that never ceases, even in deep sleep. This buzz is not 'noise', it is not meaningless activity, but it is housekeeping activity of a sort that is not obviously related to any mental activity. During the work that I am going to describe I have often sat peacefully, quite deliberately looking at the monitors showing the raw signals coming from different parts of my head, and I must say that it is a sobering experience for a brain scientist to do this. Over the screen, which has 16 channels of signals coming up on it all the time, you can see great convulsions of electrical activity spreading around, coming up like bubbles from the bottom of a pool. Yet during this whole phase, when the brain is obviously wildly boiling away and doing all sorts of electrically interesting things, one is not aware, as the subject, of thinking anything abnormal – and nothing that one thinks about makes any difference to what one sees going on on the screen.

So any idea that all one might have to do is make the head electrically transparent and immediately be able to read off what is happening in the mind would be over-optimistic. The relation between the electrical activity that *is* correlated with mental activity and the rest of the ongoing electro-encephalogram is still very obscure and as much as 99 per cent random looking. Now that is probably a reflection of our present ignorance; but I don't want to give you the idea that all one needs is a good set of amplifiers and one can automatically do mind reading. This is an impression you might otherwise get from the sort of detail that I shall go on to report.

Although the technique goes back to the 1920s, it is only since computers have allowed us to average repeated samples of brain activity under reasonably similar conditions, that we have been able to get good correlations, because these wild fluctuations, that have nothing to do with what we are interested in, can average out.

The Bereitschaftspotential: *a correlate of preparation for action*

One of the early findings of great interest in this field was that of the German physiologists, Kornhuber and Deecke in the late 1960s and early 1970s. They instructed a subject – off his own bat and with no external cues at all – to move a finger to press a button whenever he felt disposed to do so. They recorded the EEG signals continuously and delayed them so that they had a few seconds worth in a store, and as soon as the button was pressed (or as soon as the muscle activity was recorded corresponding to the movement), they triggered an averager which took out of the store the sample that was time-locked to the moving of the finger. Then they added these samples up for a couple of hundred occasions of moving the muscle and obtained an electrical profile which was repeatable, significant.

What Kornhuber and Deecke found was that up to a second before the muscle moved one could detect a steady rise in the (negative) potential over the vertex of the head. (It is the large upward wave in figure 6.1, p. 124.) They called it the *Bereitschaftspotential* (the 'preparation' or 'readiness' potential) and it is one of the landmark concepts in this field because it showed that the conscious intention to move a muscle without any external stimulus, the voluntary movement of the muscle by conscious intention, had a correlate in the brain which could be physically measured and which had its origin up to a second before the movement. Maybe this doesn't strike you as puzzling and maybe it should not have struck anyone as puzzling but there was a bias among physiologists to suppose that if a muscle moves you ought not to see anything happening except in the *motor* cortex (i.e. somewhat forward of the vertex).

What Kornhuber and Deecke had shown was that this was not the case. In a very crude sense the *intention* to move a muscle finds itself physically represented ahead of time in the potentials you can pick up, if you average long enough, over the vertex of the head.

Sir John Eccles, whom I mentioned earlier as one who calls himself a dualist interactionist and who regards the mind as occupying another 'world', regards this as crucial evidence for the action of the mind on the body, because, he says, there is no external stimulus, but here is a physical event happening long before the muscle movement which the physiologist can quantify.

I would like to suggest that the question is at least open. For it is easy to think of feedback systems which reach a threshold and trigger off an action without requiring additional instructions from outside. If you want a crude example – forgive the crudity! – think of a self-flushing toilet. The tank sits there on the wall with water dribbling in and eventually the ball that is floating on it reaches some level and lifts the valve and the water flushes out. The flow diagrams we have been drawing in earlier chapters are re-entrant flow diagrams. They characteristically do not wait on a stimulus from outside in order to initiate action. They can derive their stimulus for action from their own internal workings. Given this, it does seem to many of us that the evidence of Kornhuber and Deecke, striking though it was, can be interpreted simply as evidence that some internal process (some internal evaluator of how long it was since the last muscle movement or something like that) had simply reached threshold and provided the internal stimulus to trigger off the movement. The 'water tank' kind of model with suitable elaboration would, I think, fit well enough the evidence that the potentials that forecast a voluntary movement can be detected for up to a second before the movement occurs.

Brain correlates of preparation, evaluation and attention

The sort of thing that we have been doing at Keele is to monitor brain activity during various types of 'target practice'. On a computer screen we have a simplified 'space invader' type of game. A little square comes in from left or right. Normally the subject has to press a button so as to fire a missile at what he judges to be the right moment in order to hit the target. As soon as he presses the button the target becomes invisible but when the missile reaches the height of the target a little dash appears at the fixation point on the screen giving the subject feedback as to whether he has succeeded or not. The exact shape of the dash is slightly different for success and failure.

So we have three phases: estimation, action and evaluation. Throughout the experiment the subject fixates a prescribed spot on the screen. During the first phase, *estimation*, he sees the target coming

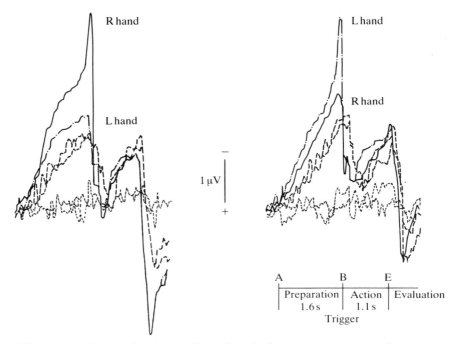

Figure 6.1 Source density profiles of evoked responses over supplementary motor areas $2\frac{1}{2}$ cm to left and right of vertex during 3.5 seconds of target practice: A, appearance of target 5 degrees to left or to right of fixation point; B, button press, which launches missile and triggers averaging computer; E, appearance at fixation point of indication of success or failure. The continuous and chain dotted traces are averages of 320 shots using right or left thumb; dashes and dots indicate the conditions 'willing' and 'staring' (see text). For these latter conditions the results are divided into two groups of 320 runs to show repeatability. (MacKay et al., 1986.)

from left or right. He judges the moment at which he ought to fire. *Action*: he presses the button. *Evaluation*: he receives the feedback and registers the outcome as success or failure.

Our question was: can we see, in different locations over the head, any electrical evidence of preoccupation with the three phases of this mental activity? The entire scalp was monitored by repeating the whole experiment five times with a net of 20 electrodes. A simplified sample of the results from just two out of 40 locations is given in figure 6.1. The traces show the electrical profile over a period of $3\frac{1}{2}$ seconds of game playing. The experiment was run at three different levels of involvement of the subject in the game. To begin with, the subject played normally using either his right or his left thumb to press the button (continuous lines and chain dots respectively). The dashed and the dotted lines are for the further conditions described below as 'willing' and 'staring'.

The results are from the area over the two supplementary motor areas, about $2\frac{1}{2}$ cm to left and right of the centre of the top of the head. This is the area where Kornhuber and his colleagues found strong signals of 'readiness' to move a muscle. You see that the potential rises until the button is pressed, and as soon as the button is pressed, the potential collapses. Then you get another rise during the second waiting period when the feedback is expected. When the feedback occurs a second big drop occurs. ('Drop' means positive-going with the sign convention here used.) You notice that the profiles are similar on the two sides of the head, except that when the right hand is used the peak is higher on the left and when the left hand is used the potential is higher on the right. That corresponds to the fact which we noticed earlier that movement of the right half of the body is controlled from the left half of the brain and vice versa.

First control experiment: 'willing'   In the first version of the experiment the subject pressed the button himself; in the second (dashes) he was invited to be a spectator while the computer fired the shots. He didn't press the button, but he was asked to interpret what was going on, to decide mentally when he thought the button ought to be pressed, and mentally to evaluate the outcome as a cheering spectator would, feeling satisfaction if the outcome was successful and disappointed if it was not. Although the potentials are smaller than those when he pressed the button himself, the resemblance is striking, provided that he was imaginatively joining in the game. The main difference is that the drop in potential is late by a few hundred milliseconds. But this is, after all, what one would expect because, whereas the actual player (in the first experiment) is the determinant of when his thumb pressed the button, the spectator can only know that the button has been pressed by seeing the missile take off. (For each of the two control conditions two separate batches of 320 shots apiece are superimposed so that one can check how reliable the results are.)

Second control experiment: 'staring'   You might well ask, how far are these potentials related to the mental activity of the subject and how far are they simply an indication that signals are coming in through the eyes? To test this the subject was asked to fixate the middle of the screen as usual but to ignore the significance of the events on the screen by occupying himself mentally in counting backwards in threes from 999. The result is the traces with small dots in figure 6.1. As you see, when attention is withdrawn, the underlying brain generates practically nothing of the earlier profile. Here we have evidence of a direct correlation between the degree of attention and the degree of electrical activity that is recordable.

Obviously we are not here in a no stimulus situation; there is a stimulus, although the moment, *t*, at which the subject decides to press the button is a matter of judgement based on earlier experience, and not simply a response to a flash of light or other command. The question is: can we go over to mental tasks which are even more covert and still find electrical correlates?

Localized brain activity during covert mental activity

Quite a lot of work on covert mental activity has been done by people who wanted to look at the difference between activity in the right and left halves of the brain. The late Professor Richard Jung, famous neurophysiologist of Freiburg in Germany, quite recently published a very interesting study. He had a subject look at a Necker cube and then deflect his attention from it by thinking of names of cities in Germany beginning with a particular letter of the alphabet. While doing this the subject continued to fixate the screen and the Necker cube, but took his mind off the input. Jung and his collaborators showed that there was, at the change of mental activity, a change, on the average, in the potential difference between the left and right sides of the head. He suggested that we might use our equipment in Keele to look at this with a finer toothed comb, as it were, not just to compare left and right but to ask whereabouts in the head the activity is going on when things like Necker cubes are either attended to or ignored.

This is a tricky experimental situation because you can't command a subject to go into a *neutral* state for comparison, all you can do is to command him to go from one mental task to another. What we have done is to choose a large number of different initial and final states.

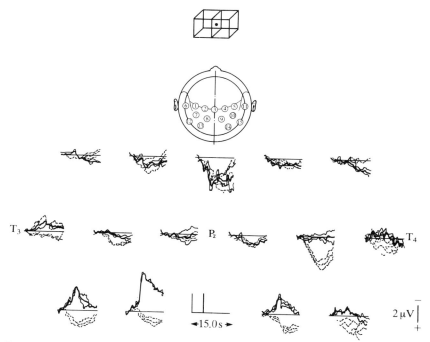

Figure 6.2   Changing one's thoughts: the change from words to Necker cube is compared with the change from words to arithmetic. Potentials across the rear of the head during two experiments in which the subject switched his thoughts (at a tone beep marked by the vertical line on the scale) from a first task to a second task. For the first experiment (continuous lines) task A was to think of words commencing with a certain letter; task B, attend to the Necker cube. For the second experiment (dotted lines) task A was again to think of words commencing with a certain letter; task B, perform mental arithmetic. For each experiment separately the grand average is shown in the heaviest print. The results are also shown divided into two batches (printed lighter) to allow reproducibility of the potentials to be judged. The electrode array had a 6 cm spacing.

(Also, in order to diminish any potentials which might be associated purely with the changeover of task irrespective of what the task was, we ran each pair of tasks in the order A, B and then B, A and subtracted the results.)

The first sample (figure 6.2, continuous traces) is one where I was first thinking of words beginning with A, until a tone sounded, when I went over to paying attention to the Necker cube so that it flipped from one perspective to the other. In the next 15 second period I thought of words beginning with B, and then switched to thinking about the Necker cube. (The Necker cube was fixated throughout both tasks.) This was repeated many times, with the computer building up an average as I worked through the alphabet. Then the same thing was done in reverse order and the results were subtracted and plotted. Two repeat batches of experiments have their results superimposed (the thin black lines) so that you can judge how well they repeat.

Then there was a second experiment (figure 6.2, dotted traces) in which, having thought of words beginning with particular letters as before, I switched, at the tone signal, to doing mental arithmetic (subtracting threes, adding sevens – the task was varied quite widely). The question is: what happens if we compare the distribution of potentials over the head during these different pairs of tasks, and more particularly upon the switching from one task to the other?

[*Interest focuses not on the* level *of the potentials, which is arbitrary, but on the direction and magnitude of the step of potential when the subject switches activity. Comparison of the two experimental conditions is therefore what we particularly look at.*] You see in figure 6.2 that there are some regions on the head where the potential actually switches in the opposite direction when you go in the one case from thinking of words to thinking of the Necker cube, and in the other case from thinking of words to mental calculation. Notice the big contrast at location 10 (right parietal), where there is practically no change in signal in the Necker case, but a huge signal in the calculation case. So mental arithmetic has its own electrical signature which is quite different from that which goes with the perceiving of the flips of the Necker cube. Then at location 13 (left occipital) there is a huge signal in the words/Necker case but only a rather small signal of the opposite polarity in the case of words/calculation. At location 3 (near vertex on midline) there is a region where the signals are the same for both pairs of tasks. So parts of the brain don't care; other parts are strongly related in their activity to the one task or the other.

In figure 6.3 we have results from somewhat further forward on the head from another subject performing the first experiment as described above, but with a different task B in the second experiment. This task we call 'map thinking'. It consists in thinking one's way around one's house, or local road system or town centre; in other

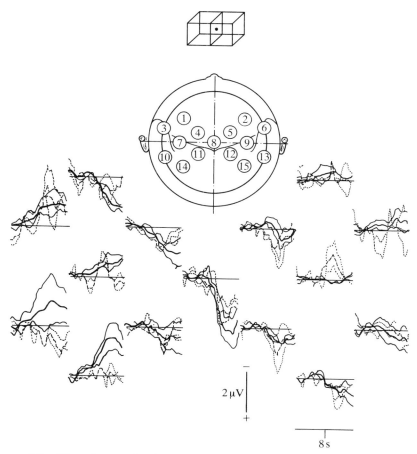

Figure 6.3 Changing one's thoughts: words to 'Necker' versus words to 'maps'. Potentials at the sides and crown of the head during two experiments in which the subject switched his thoughts. The first experiment (continuous lines) was as for figure 6.2: i.e. task A, think of words commencing with a certain letter; task B, attend to the Necker cube. For the second experiment (dotted lines), task A was again to think of words commencing with a certain letter; task B, 'map thinking'. For each experiment the results are also shown divided into two batches to show the reproducibility of the potentials. The electrode array had a 5 cm spacing.

words geographical recollecting. The electrode array is some 5 to 6 cm further forward on the head than for the previous subject. Again there is a quite different distribution of activity according to the tasks. At

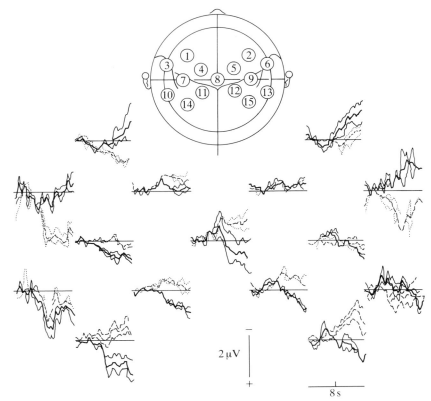

Figure 6.4 Changing one's thoughts between imaginary stimuli. Potential changes over the top of the head during two experiments in which the subject switched his thoughts. In the first experiment (continuous lines), task A was listening for a faint sound; task B was imagining the Necker cube. For the second experiment (dotted lines), task A was to listen as before; task B was to imagine a face. For each experiment the results are also shown divided into two batches to show the reproducibility of the potentials. The electrode array had a 6 cm spacing.

location 9, some 6 cm to the right of the crown of the head, the 'Necker cube thinking' produces practically no change from thinking of names, whereas map thinking produces a large change, but we notice that in this subject there is a nearly symmetrical large change produced by the switch to map thinking on the left of the head at location 7. Over on the left at locations 1 and 14, map thinking produces little effect, but viewing the Necker cube and making it flip produces a large effect. At the crown of the head, location 8, the two sets of tasks have a similar effect.

One point to emphasize, then, is that it is not a simple matter of left brain being used for one kind of task and right brain for the other; the easy popular story to that effect is much over-simplified. It is also, I think, important to realize that even in what might seem rather simple mental tasks, we have got evidence here that we are not simply stirring up one little nest of nerve cells, it is not that we have little lockers in our heads which open for particular tasks. It is a cooperative process involving many areas simultaneously.

Finally I thought I would put in figure 6.4 because the task is a purely imaginary one! The subject has to imagine two visual stimuli which he has previously seen a great deal, but which are no longer present on the empty screen. One is the double Necker cube, the other is a little circular face which darts its eyes around so that you can attend to whether you are being looked at or not. In previous experiments the subject had viewed for hours a composite picture in which face and Necker cube were simultaneously visible, so that the face seemed to be peering through the bars of a cage which was actually the Necker cube. If one fixated the nose in the middle, one could switch attention from the face and its direction of gaze to the Necker cube and its flipping of perspective. One gets very nice changes of potential while performing these two tasks, but in figure 6.4 the task was to watch a blank screen and to imagine either the face with its eyes or the Necker cube reversing. In each case task A was to listen for a very faint noise from a loudspeaker in the sound-proofed room. Imagining one or other of the visual stimuli was task B. What we find is huge differences between the results for the imagined Necker cube (black) and the imagined face (dotted). (Again we have two independent blocks of results superimposed for each experiment so that the repeatability can be seen.)

So over the scalp one can pick up localized indications of the presumed underlying brain activity correlated with imagining-a-face, which has quite a different map from the electrical activity correlated with imagining-a-Necker-cube. We did not really expect so strong a result. Both tasks are visual and yet there is no visual input, so it is a rather strongly deprived brain that is being asked to operate, but as you see the correlates are strikingly and consistently different.

Do we 'control' our brains?

Now we ought to take stock. The purpose in going through this evidence in some detail is to ask ourselves what bearing it has on the general perspective on brain–mind relations. Can we conclude from this anything relevant to the debate over the relations between brain and mind?

It is clear that mental activity here shows itself to be *efficacious*. Somebody is thinking and there are changes not merely in bodily movements, but also in small scale physical activity within his head. So you could say this is evidence that thinking, mental activity generally, has a strong causal connection with brain activity. But this is just the point at which I think we ought to pause and ask ourselves how much we want to claim here. Do we want to claim, for example, that 'we control our brains'? People often have written in these terms. Do we want to argue from this evidence, or any other, that we can have a model of the person in which the 'mind' controls the brain, which controls the muscles?

We control what we can evaluate

I would like to suggest that that would be going much further than we need. Think again of the simple case of a thermostat. What does the thermostat control? It controls the temperature; it controls that which it evaluates. Does it control its own comparator? Of course not! It is in and through the functioning of the comparator that we have a thermostat – whose capacity is to control its field of action. So control is a relation between an agent and its field of action. Controlling, I am suggesting, is a particular kind of action – action under evaluation (at least in principle). What you cannot evaluate you cannot control. To try to argue that the agent controls that in which it is itself embodied is a philosophical blunder. The agent does its evaluating in and through the activity of the evaluator. The agent determines the form of the activity but it doesn't have to control its evaluator.

What we control is what we can *evaluate*. We control our hand movements in drawing because we can evaluate the hand movements, in principle. We control our own behaviour. We can even, to some extent, control electrical signals from our heads (provided they are displayed to us as wiggles on a screen or sounds from by a microphone). For example, it is well known that people can control the firing of their own motor neurons. If suitably wired up they can hear a rattle of sound (even when the muscle does not itself move) corresponding to the nerve impulses and they can, as it were, screw themselves up mentally and somehow discover by trial and error what to do (mentally) in order to bring that rattle down.

Our ability to control that input does not, however, imply that when we are going about our normal mental business we are controlling the nerve cells in and through which our mental activity takes place. We should certainly not jump to the conclusion that this justifies a model of the brain–mind relation in which we control our brains. In general the brain activity in and through which we *do* our evaluating – in and through which our evaluating is embodied – is not something which we can control, because there is no means of evaluating it.

Range of control

What we do control is events in our domain of action within the limits of our repertoire and not outside. We can give concrete meaning to this in terms of the thermostat. The thermostat can control the temperature of a room within limits determined by the size of the heater and so forth. There are other temperatures that would be outside its control. If, for example, it was freezing cold outside and you had only a small heater, then opening the door might put the temperature of the field of action, F, outside the range of control. So there is a definite meaning to the concept of events or states *outside the control* of a given system. This will be important when we come back to the question of how far our world is outside or within our control. So mental activity, I am suggesting, determines the form of brain activity but we don't have to assume, and we do not have any grounds for saying, that it *controls* brain activity in general – although it controls the behavioural consequences of that brain activity.

No physical 'gap' is needed for mental activity to be efficaceous

You might still argue that I have not been allowing for any gaps in the physical chain of cause and effect. None of these experiments has presupposed that there would be any such gaps. So in what sense could there be any kind of efficacy in mental activity? Aren't we in danger of drifting back into epiphenomenalism where, you remember, T. H. Huxley argued that mental activity was no more causally efficacious than the steam whistle sound coming from a locomotive?

Here we have got to come back, I think, to the point about logical relativity which I made at the end of the previous chapter. We have been talking of the external world and the world of facts generally as represented in the organizing system of the brain in terms of the state of conditional readiness for action in the world. If a change takes place in the world which is relevant to the planning of action in the world, then the organizing system ought to incorporate constraints and enablements which reflect the change that has occurred in the world. In that sense the state of conditional readiness of the organizing system can be regarded as an implicit representation of what the agent *believes to be the case*.

It follows from that, as I pointed out at the end of the last chapter, that there is a physical cost in knowing and believing. A physical change has to take place in this little bit of the physical world, the organizing system inside your head, for any change that takes place in what you believe. It follows directly from that, in one line, that there cannot (logically cannot) exist a complete account of the immediate future of your state of conditional readiness which you would be correct to believe and mistaken to disbelieve. This is because your believing or disbelieving would be a material factor in its correctness. Its correctness would be determined in part by whether or not you believed it. Therefore it could not have an *unconditional* claim to your assent. Indeed on the contrary it has a built-in 'disclaim' to your assent. This notion of a disclaim to assent, i.e. a label attached saying 'not beliefworthy by X', is a crucial notion.

Out of the whole physical world, in this respect, your brain is unique. Every other state of the physical world can, in principle – assuming the laws of physics – have a specification as to its immediate future in which various events follow from the present state which you would be correct to expect and mistaken not to. But if we allow that extreme deterministic picture to apply even to your brain, the conclusion does not follow. Even if your brain were as deterministic as a clockwork model of the classical universe, there does not exist and cannot exist a complete account of its immediate future such that if only you knew it you would be correct to believe it and mistaken to disbelieve it.

Relativity of standpoint

The belief that the outside observer is correct to have about the immediate future of your cognitive machinery (the state of conditional readiness of the organizing system) is a belief that you would be mistaken to share. What this means is that even if we had a completely physically deterministic model of the working of the whole of your cognitive and supervisory system, as we have been discussing it, and hence a view of the generation of these potentials on your head, which from an outside observer's point of view was causally complete, it would not follow that from *your* standpoint you could conclude that your thinking was not causally efficacious. Quite the contrary.

From your standpoint what you are correct to believe is something that must be different from what the outside observer believes. He and you both know that you would be mistaken to believe what *he* believes. What you are correct to believe is that the immediate future of your cognitive system including the state of conditional readiness is in part for you to determine by your thinking. Your thinking will determine what form that state of conditional readiness is about to take. And that, oddly enough (because of the relativistic situation that I have already spelt out), is not logically contradicted by the evidence from the standpoint of the outside observer that the system involved is physically determinate.

The moral, which I think is worth underlining, is that in order to settle questions of this kind we must ask: from what standpoint are you asking the question? If you are asking the question from the standpoint of the detached observer, then the answer may, for all we know, be in terms of closed chain-meshes of physical cause and effect. But if you are asking the question from the standpoint of the agent, then the observer himself, if he knows his onions, will insist that the agent would be correct to believe something else. And what he is correct to believe is not that there is 'room' in the sense of vague, wishy-washy, indeterminate, random relations between prior and later events in his mental activity, but that there are quite precise, corresponding, correlated connections between the way he thinks, evaluates and chooses and the immediate future of his state of conditional readiness. In that sense, we have not just an easy, neutral cohabitation of the deterministic outside observer's view and the voluntaristic agent's view. The two fit as neatly as hand and glove.

Notes

1 More recently (1989), by use of phosphorus rather than proton resonance, it has become possible to use magnetic resonance imaging techniques to monitor activity.

7

The Divided Brain

I want to raise three questions in this chapter which, at first sight, may seem to have little in common, but I hope by the end that you will see they are interrelated. The first is: what makes us a unity and, in particular, how far does thinking about the brain as an integrated information system help us to see what it is about our embodiment that makes us a unity? The second question is: how can we consider, for scientific purposes, what happens when two conscious agents meet and interact? If you like, how do the processes of communication and dialogue look in terms of the kind of information-flow modelling that we have been doing? And the third question is: what can we learn from human cases in which the two cerebral hemispheres of the brain have been surgically separated; the famous 'split brain' operation?

So first, what is it that makes us a unity? Now you might think that it is absurd to raise this question. Here we are, each within one skin, and you might imagine that the physical integrity of the body as an organism is enough, but as you will see by the end of the chapter, there are good grounds for doubting whether simply having all the structures together in one head would be enough to guarantee that the organism could be regarded as a unitary individual.

We saw in chapter 6 that there is a good deal of evidence – and that was only a very small sample – that different conscious activities can have physical correlates which are scattered over both hemispheres, front and back, left and right.

The left–right axis

When one looks at the overall shape of the brain one finds some evidence, though not very strong or striking, that the two halves of the brain, which we tend to think of as symmetrical, are somewhat asymmetrical. (See, for example, plate 1.) The left hemisphere is usually longer than the right and the shapes and positions of the folds and ridges differ considerably – suggesting even at that level that there are perhaps differences of function in the right and left hemisphere information-flow systems.

Let us remind ourselves of some of the other evidence. [*We have spoken already of the way that there is a pretty clear and symmetrical division along the right–left axis of sensory input from eyes and hands. This applies to the skin, the joints, the pain receptors and proprioceptors and also to the motor output to the limbs. The right half of our body and of our field of view has its processing performed in the left half brain, and the left half of our world in the right half brain. Hearing, however, and many other functions are not so sharply divided, and the olfactory signals from the two nostrils are not crossed over to the opposite hemispheres.*]

A sharp left–right divide is displayed in the striking phenomenon of 'neglect', which sometimes results when either hemisphere is damaged towards the rear in the parietal region. This is a lack of attention to, or awareness of, the entire half of the body, its clothes and surroundings on the side controlled from the damaged hemisphere. The sort of thing that occurs in some cases is illustrated by plate 20, from the work of the late Professor Richard Jung of Freiburg. He studied a painter, Anton Räderscheidt, who in October 1967 suffered damage to his right parietal area. Two years previously Räderscheidt had done a self-portrait (a) which, as you can see, does reasonable justice to both sides of his face. Then he suffered the brain damage, which led to hemianopsia (the loss of half his visual field) and also this phenomenon of neglect. He was aware of the loss of the left half of his visual field and could make up for it by moving his eyes to see wherever he wanted to; nevertheless, when he attempted a self-portrait he depicted only one side of his face (b). Five months after the brain damage in March 1968, there was considerably greater realism (d) but still a tendency to neglect the left side of his face.

Patients with this sort of trouble will also either refuse to admit or refuse to bother to describe features in the world around them on the 'missing' side. So this specialization of the hemispheres which we have already looked at in terms of normal sensory and motor function can extend also into domains which are much more closely connected with voluntary behaviour and planning and so on.

There is then, in the undamaged brain, a real question as to what it is that unifies activity on the two sides – diverse in geography and also, it seems, in character. Speech, for example, is well known to be affected more by lesions to the left hemisphere than to the right. It is, as we say, a left hemisphere function. Then there are more subtle functions, some of which are associated primarily with the right hemisphere. For example, Gestalt perception, the ability to perceive groupings of features as a single object, is more seriously impaired by damage to the right of the brain than to the left, particularly towards the back of the head.

In the literature of ten to twenty years ago there was a fairly general tendency to downgrade the right hemisphere. People spoke of the 'major' and 'minor' hemispheres, the left hemisphere, controlling speech, being supposed to be the 'major' or 'dominant' hemisphere. This perception is currently being criticized. Even within the field of speech there is evidence that right hemisphere damage, although it leaves the left hemisphere able to generate the sounds, the words, of speech, can have a serious effect on the emotional and prosodic content. In other words, it is not that the left hemisphere speaks, and the other one does other (non-speech) things. It is rather that the left hemisphere organizes the syntactic and other content of the speech, while the right hemisphere contributes to the intonation, the rise and fall of the voice and so forth.

The field is thus moving towards a position where much stronger credit is given to both hemispheres. As an example of the redressing of the balance here is part of a recent summary article by Dr Elliot Ross:

Since the fundamental discoveries that lesions in the left hemisphere cause language disorders, vast numbers of studies have delineated the linguistic and related functions of the left hemisphere and this has led to the widely held opinion that the 'dominant' or 'major' hemisphere is the left while the right is relegated to a minor or non-dominant role. During the last decade neurological and neuropsychological evidence has been gathered which shows that this point of view is incorrect, and that the true richness and complexity of human communication and behaviour is only partially represented in the left hemisphere. There is much clinical evidence that the right hemisphere has a major role in the attitudinal and emotional aspects of language through its dominant modulation of the affective components of prosody and gestures. (Ross, 1984.)

That is, the two hemispheres are seen as playing different and complementary roles. But it all leaves us still with the question: how is this whole system unified? The more you see one hemisphere as specializing in one aspect of a performance and the other as specializing in another, the more you wonder what is the basis of their unity other than mere contiguity.

The unification of the localized functions

Sir John Eccles, to whom I referred earlier as a leading dualist interactionist, says quite frankly that he sees no answer to this question other than to invoke the services of the 'mind', viewed as an entity in another world which is able to interact with the two hemispheres, and by – as he sometimes says – 'taking a look over from one hemisphere into the other', drawing together the information that is available and the coordination that is needed, on the two sides. Again I can't say that there is anything in science to disprove this, but our question now will be whether we need to go to the extreme of postulating this kind of interaction in order to perceive a basis for the unity.

What I would like to do is to exploit once more the minimally simple information-flow diagram (figure 3.2) which we have been using to represent the integrative operations of the brain as an information system. It is the minimal, most economical flow map that can bring in some of the essential features not merely of responsive activity of the sort that a thermostat can carry out, but that also can evaluate its own goal criteria and change them if necessary.

It had essentially two parts: a lower and an upper storey, so to speak, and I am going to redraw it now with a slight elaboration of the upper storey to bring out the fact that we are discussing a hierarchic state of organization (figure 7.1). At the lower level (lighter lines) we have the receptor and effector systems (R and E). As we remarked before, these are linked by a process of evaluation, or comparison

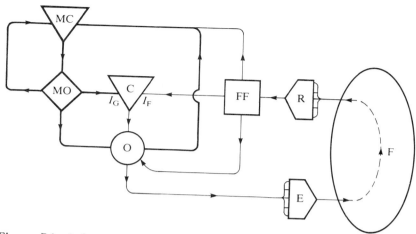

Figure 7.1 Information-flow map for a system capable of self-organized goal-directed activity, redrawn so as to bring out its essentially hierarchic nature. Heavy lines represent the supervisory or meta-organizing level. MO, meta-organizing system. The metacomparator, MC, represents one member of a hierarchy of evaluators.

(within C), of the indicated state with the goal state, leading to the organization of action (in O) calculated to bring the field into the goal state. That flow-loop is familiar to most of us in terms of a thermostat or automatic pilot.

Then we have, unchanged, the feedforward path with its feature-filters, FF. They are the things that pull out of the sensory input the clues the organizing system needs in order to keep itself up to date. They provide clues as to the appropriate state of readiness to reckon with the field. This state of readiness then comes to represent the field in the kind of way, I was suggesting, that the angle of the steering wheel of a car which has just driven up a semi-circular drive represents the curvature of the drive.

We then come to the second order process (heavy lines) which is concerned with the setting of the goals of the system. An autonomous organism requires of course to set its own goals. So we have drawn the meta-organizing system with a meta-evaluative procedure to take stock of how things are going. It adjusts or reselects the current goal in the light of its evaluation of the success of ongoing agency, and it also keeps up to date the organizing system to match the state of the world indicated by the feedforward from the receptor system.

In other words I have teased the supervisory system out into two compartments which, as you see, are each formally similar to figure 3.1. So there is a meta-organizing system, which organizes the activity in the organizing system in the way that the organizing system organizes the activity in the outside world. It includes the meta-comparator, MC, a second-order evaluative system which monitors the success of the whole system and instructs the meta-organizing system, MO, to change goal priorities if, in the light of the current criteria of higher order evaluation, that is necessary. In other words this is repeating the recipe that we already used in figure 3.1. I have drawn it like this with heavy lines to make clear that this can be regarded as the first stage of quite a large hierarchy. This process can go on from level to level so that you can evaluate the merits of changing a criterion of evaluation at a lower level. This idea, then, that the flow map (which we are tentatively adopting as a minimal thought model of the organization of conscious human agency) is *hierarchic* is quite basic.

Evaluation

The general term which we have been using for the self-regulating activity of such a feedback loop is evaluation. Evaluation is a process in which an indication of the current state is compared against a goal criterion, a norm, a priority, and the result is assessed as 'plus' or 'minus'. The comparator issues positive or negative evaluation, and on the basis of this evaluation the organizing or meta-organizing system selects action, at either the lower or the higher level, calculated to maximize positive evaluation or maintain it and remove negative evaluation. That is the information engineer's minimum skeleton for self-organized goal-directed agency. Such a system is its own programmer. It doesn't have, like a thermostat, a knob ending in free air for somebody to turn to set goals. It undertakes the task of setting its own goals and goal priorities.

Unity of our conscious agency

Our question now is: if this is taken as a summary of some of the minimal functions of the brain at this level, what constitutes *its* unity?

Now you will notice, and I emphasize this, that the receptor system is a many-channel parallel affair. Not only are there eyes and ears in parallel but also from the eyes and from the ears many signals come in in parallel. Furthermore, as we saw earlier there are many 'maps' in the brain of the external visual field; that is, there are many projections from the retina to different parts of the brain in terms of such things as texture, motion or colour. So even in such a field as perception we have many processes going on in parallel in the brain. Now we have already faced the question: what makes the perceived world a unity? My suggestion was that it is the existence of only one state of conditional readiness to reckon with the world. There is only one centralized organ for the setting up of conditional readinesses for possible action within the world which originates the sensory input.

What I am going to suggest now as our working hypothesis is that the unity of conscious agency, which we associated as its correlate particularly with the meta-organizing or self-supervisory level of this whole information-flow system, is constituted by the unity of the evaluative process at the top level.

If you ask what we are, what it is about us that distinguishes us most from sticks and stones and other objects, and contemplate the various aspects of our conscious experience, I think that the core of the answer is that we have the capacity – indeed the necessity – to *evaluate*. Our capacity to evaluate situations as positive or negative, to take stock and make plans in view of norms and priorities, is at least one of our most characteristic features and certainly one of those to which the singular term 'I' is most naturally attached: 'I want this, I like this, I dislike that, I am dissatisfied with that, this hurts me,' and so on. There is room for a lot of argument at the technical engineering level that we are also a unity as agents in the world, that our limbs and so on function with a lot of cross-checks and balances, so that they are integrated in unitary activity. But I am suggesting that, at the end of the day, what constitutes our unity is the singleness of the top level of the evaluative hierarchy which takes stock of our priorities and assesses the current state of affairs with a plus or a minus.

For the rest of this chapter we shall be considering what implications this has (if we take it as a working hypothesis), firstly for our consideration of the process of communication and secondly for the analysis and understanding of the phenomena of the split brain operation.

Communication between agents

Taking this general conception of the human organism as a self-supervisory evaluative agent, can we extract features which are particularly relevant to the process we call communication? What happens when two such systems encounter one another? In terms of our map the other individual is part of the field of action. You remember that our general idea is that the contents of the field of action, the stable contents that are worth representing for practical purposes, find themselves represented in the conditional readiness of the organizing system to bring about goal-directed action in the field. So we want to ask ourselves what kind of representation of the other, the other conscious agent, we would expect to find, we would need to have, in the organizing system of each of them if each is to perceive the other as a goal-directed agent.

Here I think it is useful to distinguish three aspects of the internal representation which the organizing system embodies. For our present purpose we can use an economical representation of some of the functions which are implicit in our flow map of figure 7.1 when considering communication between such systems. I have sketched against the three divisions of the system in figure 7.2 the terms maps, skills and norms. In doing this I have collapsed the whole of the supervisory system into the compartment that is labelled norms; the

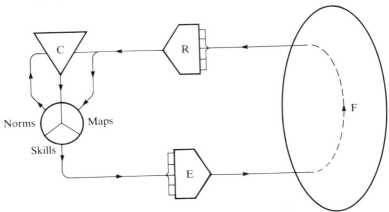

Figure 7.2 Goal-directed agent – essentials of the information-flow map of figure 7.1 for consideration of interaction between agents.

feedforward and so forth are collapsed into the compartment labelled maps, and skills represents the other types of readiness, including the readiness to write your name or speak, or things of that sort. The terms, I think are fairly self-explanatory.

'*Maps*': You have already heard me fulminate against the idea that we need little models of the world in our heads that literally are like maps. We don't need a little television screen looking like the visual world in order that we should see, and likewise for the other senses. So here 'maps', in quotes, indicates that representation, almost certainly implicit, of the layout of the world which determines our conditional readiness to navigate in the world. Under the term navigate I want to include the throwing of the eye around the world. This I think is what characterizes the internal representation of the visual world. It is a state of conditional readiness to throw the retina from point to point (through the projection mechanism of the lens). One can make a similar point for the rest of our spatial readinesses to reckon with the world. 'Maps' stands for all of that.

Skills: Skills stands for the concatenated organizations of the repertoire which are involved in speaking, handwriting, and so forth.

Norms: Norms is a label which includes the whole process of setting priorities, revising some priorities in the light of others and adopting, from time to time, new priorities on the basis of evaluation of the satisfactoriness or otherwise of those currently embodied.

Communication

The reason for going to this more economical diagram is that when we come to talk about communication and the internal representation of the other member of a dialogue, it is around these three heads (maps, skills and norms) that I think it is particularly easy to focus the business of internal representation. In figure 7.3 we simplify matters to some of the skeleton features of the way we can think about com-munication between two individuals. We have two egg-shaped objects A and B, each divided into three sectors, labelled maps, skills and norms, with everything else presupposed around these.

When two information systems representing the flow systems of two human beings are in interaction, of course there is a level at which the one can be treated as an object by the other. If all you have got to do is

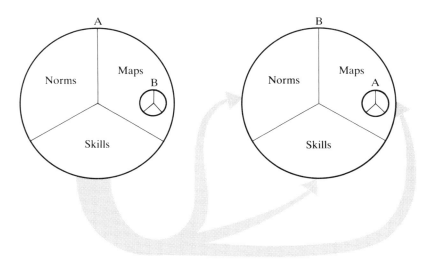

Figure 7.3   Essentials of communication by agent A to agent B.

lift people off a ferry, or something like that, then it is enough that you should represent them as a mass in your map of the world. You use your skill to do the lifting and that's all. But if you are in face with another, there is a special mode, that we all learn from infancy, in which your interaction takes the form of a skilled emission of a signal – by speech, gesture, writing or otherwise – which has a target. Its target may be any one of the three departments that we have crudely separated out in the organizing system. In other words, if we think of it in concrete terms, one of the important functions of communication (although not the whole function) is to bring up to date the map of another.

An *indicative* utterance can be thought of from this point of view as a tool, a tool designed to reach into the organizing system of the other, to get into his map section and enter a feature which otherwise would not be there. It is a substitute for perception from this point of view and it has a certain 'selective function' (we shall be using this phrase quite a bit). Its function is to select, out of all the possible map conditions or, more precisely, states of conditional readiness, one state of conditional readiness. Thus if I tell you that someone is outside the door waiting to see you, you may do nothing about it, but you have a *conditional readiness*, if you go outside the door, to expect to find him there and to talk to him. So communication, in its indicative mode, can be seen as a kind of second-hand perception: it is a way of updating the state of conditional readiness other than through the sense organs.

Of course you can then go on to other sorts of communication. Skills can be communicated by the process we call *instructive* communication. In the case of *commands* the target of the communicative utterance is the normative system. A command could take the form of a request. There are all sorts of modes of imperative communication. *Interrogative* communication is an interesting special case where what you do is to aim at the normative system. A aims at the normative system of B and seeks to set up in B the goal of bringing A up to date. So it is the beginning of a reciprocal relation. If I ask you, 'what is the time?', my statement does of course inform you, in an indicative manner, that I don't know what the time is, but I calculate it to stir in you the setting of a goal priority of updating my knowledge of the time. Normally you respond by saying 'it's nearly 6 o'clock' or whatever.

So this kind of flow model, in spite of its simplicity and crudity, finds room for many of the distinctions that we need between different types of communication.[1]

Meaning

Now what about meaning? What is the meaning of a communication in these terms? I suggest that it comes directly out in terms of the selective function of the tool which you have designed. The meaning of a statement that 'it is 6 o'clock' is its *selective function on the range of states of readiness of the recipient* for reckoning with the time. We have here the basis of a kind of anatomy of the communicative process in which you see the correlates of such distinctions as 'intended meaning', 'received meaning' and 'conventional meaning' in terms of: the selective function set up in A's normative system, the selective function actually achieved in B's appropriate system and the selective function calculated with respect to a standard ensemble of B's, i.e. the 'dictionary meaning'.

I say all this just to give you a feeling for the way in which we can extend our information-flow analysis to these more complex interactions between two and more individuals, in order to show that we can now also take stock of our question of truth, from another angle.

Truthful communication

In chapter 5 I warned that the principle of logical relativity (which seems to be quite inescapable) forces us to distinguish between the accuracy of a description and the truthfulness of the transmission of that description because transmitting a description to you of your state of conditional readiness will automatically make that description out of date and incredible for you – not merely psychologically unbelievable, but such that you would be mistaken to believe it. It is *unbelief-worthy* with a disclaim to your assent.

Now we can come back to figure 7.3 and ask what would constitute truthful communication. We see that communicating to you the current state of your internal representation of the world would necessarily be untruthful, because it would necessarily bring about a change that would make the description out of date and erroneous. That is only one form of untruthfulness (that can be very easily identified) where logic would not, as it were, constitute an automatic test. But what this approach brings out is that it is not the only one.

For instance, there are very many ways in which you can speak to somebody ironically – making only true statements as far as a logician would go, but creating an impression which is entirely false. I won't bore you with illustrations, but we all know how politicans and others can use these tricks. If, however, we adopt our present kind of engineering analysis of what *selective function is intended* by A on B's state of conditional readiness we can get hard-nosed criteria of untruthfulness which are much more trustworthy, much more realistic, and might in the end be much more devastating for this disgusting practice, than the use of logic. I say this not because I have anything against logic, but because logic is designed for the evaluation of correspondences between descriptions and states of affairs and not for the evaluation of communicative acts as such.

The reciprocity of dialogue

Finally on this score notice that in order to perceive A's action as a communication by A (rather than merely as a symptom of a state of affairs from which something might be inferred by B), B has to have

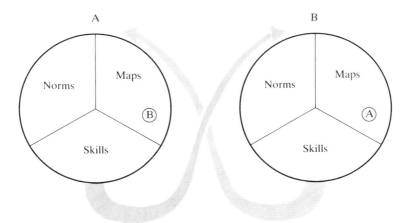

Figure 7.4   'Figure of eight' flow map for agents coupled in dialogue.

an internal representation at least of A's normative priorities in doing it (MacKay, 1972). In other words we get a very interesting reciprocal situation where B's map must include within it a little map of A; and A's map must include a little map of B. This of course results in a feedback loop, a closed loop, a re-entrant situation where the kind of logical relativity principle that I have been enunciating applies not merely to the one and to the other singly, but to the two as a joint system.

We are looking in figure 7.4 at a stylized map of the two states of conditional readiness and what we are saying is, the coupling that we call 'dialogue' – in which each perceives the other as a goal-directed communicator with the goal of reciprocally affecting the other's state of conditional readiness – this relationship of dialogue constitutes the two one information-flow system. For purposes of causal analysis, for purposes of prediction, for anything else, the two that are reciprocally coupled in dialogue are one system.

I suggest that we have, in the presence of this curious 'figure of eight' flow map of information, the correlate of the (I think to all of us) unique experience of being in dialogue with someone else. We all know the difference it makes at Madame Tussaud's, if you go up to what you take to be a waxwork figure and poke it in the belly, and discover that you are in the presence of another centre of awareness like yourself. The closing of the loop is almost palpably felt in that situation. Part of the mystery – and it is a genuine mystery and not a bogus one – of what it is to experience dialogue with another, and to share, in some sense, with the other the experience of being a centre of awareness, comes, I think, through the fact that while you are in dialogue with the other you are *one information system*. The fact that there are links that are not fleshly, through the eyes or the ears or whatever, from the information engineer's standpoint doesn't matter – he's accustomed to using satellites as part of his information systems! The experience then of indwelling, of one information system being constituted of two, could be expected to have something subjectively unique about it and I suggest that indeed it does.

[*Two further illustrations are added below.*]

Negotiation

Becoming one system does not, of course, mean sharing a single set of norms. There are the special situations of marriage or of playing instruments together (these are examples of dialogue in the sense in which Martin Buber used the word) where it has been agreed that the process of norm-setting shall be so tightly coupled as to be joint. But in general the kind of coupling that we have in figure 7.4 does not prevent A's normative system from remaining independent of B's. Think for example of two negotiators; they may have very different priorities embodied implicitly in their normative systems but of course they want to form as accurate an impression as they can of one another's normative priorities to interact in a goal *conflict* situation.

The art of dialogue can be spelt out as the art of securing enough goal compatibility for mutual advantage. Think of the simple model of two air-conditioners sharing a room but with their thermostats set to incompatible temperatures. What is going to happen? Well, they will both run flat out, one heating, one cooling and one or other of them is going to burn itself out quite soon. However, if one of them by accident or design is able to send out a hand which turns the other's knob into coincidence with its own they both settle down to sharing the load and they live for ever after each bearing half the load that they would otherwise have had to carry. That is a simple example of the use of communication to readjust norms and I would say that is the case between normal individuals in dialogue.

Representation of another

[*It may be asked, in the figure of eight situation where A has a map of B and B has map of A (figure 7.4), whether either of them can ever have an accurate internal representation of the other.*] This is indeed a good question. If you are not careful, the attempt to inform yourself fully of the condition of someone who is reciprocally trying to inform himself fully on you can go unstable. You can get neurotic situations developing in families sometimes which have some hint of resemblance to that kind of situation. The answer is to rest content with a more sketchy representation of the other. Even in the situation of the TV and its camera which we looked at in chapter 1, if the camera had focused in on a single pixel then the instability could have settled down. This is something we all learn in our interactions with one another: the difference between a decent interaction in which you represent the other in skeleton form and the kind of interaction which, if you insisted on pursuing it, might drive the other individual, or both of you, crazy is perhaps analogous to that.

[*Two people approaching a glass door from opposite sides offer a familiar situation in which each agent is forming a picture of the world which includes the other. The more either of them tries to be sensitive to exactly what the other is about to do, the more he is receiving signals which include reactions to what he himself appears to be doing or intending to do.*] So, yes, A's representation of B must always be an underspecified representation, and B's of A must be underspecified, because there does not exist one and only one representation of B, including his representation of A, which could be complete in detail with a claim to A's assent.

Communities

Don't let us be misled by the syllable 'di-' in the word dialogue. It doesn't of course mean only an interaction between two people. Dialogue means mutual transparency. All the points I have been making apply, with suitable modifications, to all members of a community in dialogue.

For all the members of a community in dialogue the standpoint is a common one from the relativistic angle. That is to say, all of them together would equally be mistaken to accept the kind of account which the outside observer, who tells the brain story in our parable, could correctly believe about them. More of that when we come to discuss responsibility.

Higher mental functions

Once this skill of moulding the conditional readinesses of another has developed it is also capable, in the human being at least, of being turned upon the system itself. The skill of talking to someone else can be employed (the same subroutines in the state of conditional readiness mechanism can be employed) on one's *own* conditional readiness. So one has all the advantages of the highly sophisticated tool construction which develops for purposes of persuading other people, raising questions with other people, and so forth, in getting to work on one's own internal organizing system. This, I think, may be the correlate of what are called 'higher mental functions'. Higher mental functions would in this sense be parasitic on the practice of communication.

And of course we are not just talking about verbal communication. We are talking about the sort of thing that starts in the nursery at the breast – all the reciprocities which gradually build up between an infant and its personal environment contribute to the internal repertoire which can be turned upon the business of revising one's own internal state of conditional readiness, making anticipatory experiments, running as we would say 'imaginary scenarios', to see how it might turn out. All of these things can make heavy and profitable use of the repertoire of skills developed for the art of communication with others.

'Split brain' phenomena

The brain, as we have seen in plates 1 and 2, looks rather like a walnut with its two halves connected by several structures, particularly the massive linking cableway of the corpus callosum which contains millions of cross-connecting fibres. In plate 17, which is a front to back section through the middle of the 'walnut', the corpus cal-

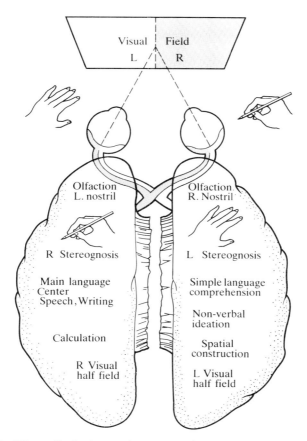

Figure 7.5 The split brain syndrome: a schematic summary of the functional lateralization evident in behavioural tests of patients with forebrain commissurotomy. The signals from and to each hand and from the left and right halves of each retina are processed in the opposite hemisphere. With the corpus callosum cut, the information in each cerebral hemisphere is not directly accessible to the other hemisphere. (Sperry, 1968.)

losum is the large white curved feature, its fibres running perpendicular to the plane of the page.

In a small number of patients the corpus callosum has been cut (and often also the smaller anterior commisure) because they had intractable epilepsy generated in one half of the brain and spreading over those fibres to the other half. This operation provides them with enough relief to make the loss of coherence of the two halves acceptable.

Roger Sperry and others used patients in this condition to make tests whose results are summarized in figure 7.5, which is from one of their early papers. When a 'split brain' patient is invited to look at the middle of a screen (marked 'visual field' in the figure) the information from the right half of the visual field, and of the body, is projected to the left hemisphere and the information from the left half of the world goes to the right half brain, as in all of us. But without the corpus callosum neither cerebral hemisphere has access to the information in the other, so various functions are separated in these patients as indicated. The main speech organizing system (or 'language centre', as it is called in this old picture) is on the left. [*The capacity to control fine finger positions in each hand and also to interpret touch information from them is confined to the hemisphere opposite to the hand. The following experiment is typical of many which contributed to this summary picture.*]

The patient looks at the dot in the middle of the screen, and the word KEY is flashed on the left and simultaneously the word RING on the right. [(*The reason for flashing the visual information onto the screen for only 100 ms is to prevent the patient from having enough time to move the eyes and receive all the information in both halves of the retina and thus in both halves of the brain.*)]

KEY . RING

The patient is asked verbally: 'please retrieve from the objects which you can feel on the table in front of you' (hidden behind a little curtain) 'whatever has been named on the screen'. In the above case the patient retrieved a key with the left hand and a ring with the right but when the patient was asked 'what word did you see on the screen?', he replied 'I saw ring', and denied having seen key; at least his mouth denied it. There is a great deal of evidence of this sort, on the basis of which Sperry has spoken of these patients as having 'two free wills in the one cranial vault'.

Now we shall be discussing free will several times, but at the very least I would like to suggest that in order to maintain that we are in a situation with two free wills there ought to be two independent *evalua-tive hierarchies*, or at least two independent ultimate evaluators. My wife and I were offered, very kindly, facilities by Sperry to test some of his patients and later we tested some of Gazzaniga's to see how far the evidence justified believing that the operation of callosotomy had in effect set up two rival and independent centres of ultimate evaluation of priorities, as distinct from organizing systems with independent sensori-motor programs.

The evidence is quite clear that the two sensori-motor programs *are* independent. In fact one of the first things we did was to try out a test of the following sort:

ADD   ADD

2 . 4
1   0

This is a task of simultaneous arithmetic; the left hand side gets one little sum, and the right a different one (you can also have adding on the one side and subtracting on the other). The numerical answer is always in the range nought to five. Fix the eye on the dot in the middle of the little square on the computer screen; the words ADD and/or SUBTRACT are steadily present; two numbers come up briefly on either side. The patient was asked to show the answer by extending fingers on each hand (a clenched fist was to signify nought). The patient's hands are under a cloth, out of sight for the subject, but not for the experimenters. The patients obtained scores on this which fell in the middle of our range of results from normals and their left hands did nearly as well as their right. So in the patients it seemed that both halves of the patient were almost equally able to perform these simple arithmetical tasks. [*It was noticeable that they all took the task in their stride whereas many normals reeled under the general sense of memory overload and fleeting impressions. One patient, VP, for many minutes calmly produced near perfect scores on both hands when adding in one half field and subtracting in the other.*]

There were many other experiments of this kind to show that in this sense the levels of sensori-motor and goal-directed activity had been split by the operation. You could in this way say that there are two 'wills': there are two targets, there are two goals on the two sides. We had one experiment, for example, in which we arranged that the subject had to move two levers with one finger of each hand to bring arrows into line with numerals on a scale according to numbers that had been flashed. This they were able to do very easily with their fingers. I then meanly and without notice mechanically locked the two levers together. One subject actually wrenched the lock round with the two hands so as to force the arrows on the screen to the appropriate numerals. This was thus a definite physical struggle between the two half systems. Call this, if you like, a 'conflict of will'. But if you think about it, suppose you were an organist who wanted to pull out one stop on the organ and to push another one in and some goat like me were to go behind the scenes and lock the two together. What would the organist do? He would pull hard on the one and push on the other. This provides no evidence whatever that he is a split person; simply that he has indeed a different programme with a different target for his left hand and his right. So our tentative judgement as far as that was concerned was that it shows simply that at the lowest level of our organizing hierarchy you can have independent goal settings for independent subdepartments of the effector system.

But the question that I put to Sperry and that took us out to California was whether we could, if Sperry was right, give a split brain patient the experience of meeting his other half in dialogue. This is why I have gone into the matter of dialogue first. Could we set up the kind of reciprocal relationship that would be called dialogue between two different centres of awareness – between two 'free wills', if you like. We tried very hard: we tried getting the halves of the patients to play games like noughts and crosses against each other (without their realizing that they were their own adversary) but found this disappointing. One famous patient, NG, was not a noughts and crosses strategist, and another, LB, had developed over the 15 years since his operation so many ways of 'cross-cueing' – that is, of giving himself clues on the one side by way of his neck proprioceptors, vestibular system and other ways, as to what information had come in on the other – that that didn't work out. Later, to cut a long story short, we were in New York with one of Gazzaniga's recent patients, JW, whose brain is known from NMR scans to be well split (anterior commisure in addition to corpus callosum). He is a cheerful person and was very happy to engage in a game of a different sort.

'Twenty questions'

We trained JW's speaking half to cross-question me about a mystery number, which I knew but he didn't. I answered his (verbal) questions by pointing to a card on which were the words 'go up', 'go down' and 'OK'. So the speaking half became able to play the 'twenty questions' game speedily and skilfully. We then trained the non-speaking half to point to the card to give me information as to whether *my* guesses needed to go up or down to find a digit that the non-speaking half (i.e. left visual field) had seen but I had not. So each half patient was trained to play a different role in the game of twenty questions. Then we said, how about playing this game yourself? So we flashed a number to the non-speaking half (and a word or picture as 'distractor' to the right). We verified that the mouth was unable to bear witness to what the digit was on the left hand side of the visual field. Then we said 'now guess'. And the mouth would guess. I always had to say 'left hand answer'. It didn't run freely. But provided I said 'left hand answer', the left hand would come out and point correctly to 'go up' or 'go down'. Suppose for example the mystery digit was seven. The mouth might guess 'nine'; the left hand would point to 'go down'; the mouth might guess 'five'; the left hand would point to 'go up'; the mouth would say 'seven' and the left hand pointed to 'OK' and the patient would smile.

So we had a satisfactory interchange of information between the two halves. But still the question was: what about the priority determining level? Can we get cross-bargaining going between the two sides – a struggle of will, in other words – rather than a mere exchange of indicative information? To this end we introduced rewards. We had an open box of tokens for each hand and a system of rewards and penalties in which the left hand was rewarded by the speaking half for each answer it gave. Without boring you with details, this game proceeded smoothly for some time.

Then we introduced the opportunity for two 'free wills' to show themselves – if there were two free wills there – by suggesting that the left hand might like to determine the level of reward by pointing to a card on which the numbers 1, 2 and 3 were written. The left hand immediately pointed to '3' (tokens per answer), wanting the biggest possible reward. The game proceeded, but the right side was speedily bankrupted by this immoderate demand for reward. So we raised the question of whether the left hand would settle for less. The left hand pointed to the numeral '2' but the mouth synchronously said 'sure, settle for less'. This of course was a negative result so it is not a conclusive proof. But it seemed to us that having given the best possible opportunity for a duality of will, a separation, an independence of norm-setting activity to show itself, the situation did not reveal any sign of the sort of conflict of will that two rival centres of awareness might have shown. Indeed JW said (quite good humouredly, because he was enjoying all this): 'What are you guys trying to do: make two people out of me?'

Conclusions from the split brain evidence

Taking stock of all the evidence that has so far been published on the duality of goal directedness which you undoubtedly find in split brain patients, I am not aware of any, including these experiments that my wife and I did, which justify one in saying that there are 'two free wills in the one cranial vault'. And you will ask me, what then is the alternative way of describing what is happening, because there is a pretty severe separation of something? One can certainly say that these are individuals who can be, and often are, 'in-two-minds'. I would plead that we leave the hyphens in! I am not saying they *have* two minds: I am saying they are in-two-minds. We sometimes use that expression about ourselves. We can be torn between alternatives, we can even sometimes get ourselves into a semi-neurotic condition in which our spoken instructions to others, for instance, may be at odds with what our hands are trying to bring about because we have not solidly settled which of two possible paths we are pursuing. And I think there is evidence that these unfortunate people can be more seriously in-two-minds and have less insight, be less aware of the kind of duality that has overtaken their goal-level setting process, than normal individuals who have the communicative pathways between the hemispheres intact. (One hope that one has while interacting with the patients is that one may give them insight into ways in which they can help themselves by cross-cueing.)

But I would say that the idea that you can create two individuals merely by splitting the organizing system at the level of the corpus callosum which links the cerebral hemispheres is unwarranted by any of the evidence so far. It is also in a very important sense implausible. I say this with hindsight because there was a time when I think the brain science fraternity generally accepted the idea that because the most distinctive development in *Homo sapiens*, compared with other animals, was at the level of the cerebral cortex, the cortex must be the organ of consciousness and *the* site of what makes man distinctive. Now as regards the capacity to cross-correlate and detect covariations, and so on, we have had plenty of evidence that that is likely to be the case. But to conclude from this that the location of what we have been calling the 'top level' of the evaluative hierarchy is cortical, seems to me to be quite unwarranted. Indeed there is evidence that many of the deep structures of the nervous system, which are not separated in the operation that Sperry and others have studied, are more closely linked with deep priorities – emotional states and things of that sort – than are the cortical areas. And certainly there are a number of operations that can damage or remove huge areas of cortex without abolishing conscious experience. They abolish or confuse the components of conscious experience that would have been contributed to by the part of the cortex removed, but you don't render the patients unconscious even by removing an entire cerebral hemisphere. So my own guess – purely on the clinical evidence and in line with Penfield's instincts – is that the centro-encephalic system and other appendages may be the physical basis of norm-setting, and the extent to which that could be split and still function is rather doubtful.

We can crudely picture the human central nervous system as a structure shaped like a capital Y, but with the corpus callosum normally forming a bridge between the upper ends of the Y, which of course represent the two cerebral hemispheres. Multiple pathways are known to run in both directions along all three arms of the Y. If the only direct correlate of conscious experience were cortical activity, then it would be plausible that cutting the corpus callosum should bring two separate 'streams of consciousness' into being. If, however, as I am arguing, the physical correlate of our conscious experience is likely to be the cooperative to-and-fro traffic between cortical and deeper levels of neural activity (i.e. levels below the junction of the two arms), then although removal of the callosal bridge could be expected to bring separate left and right executive systems into being, it would give no reason to doubt the continued unity of the conscious person. It is only if the neural equipment for self-supervisory normative activity were known to be completely duplicated (in *each* hemisphere) at cortical levels normally linked by the corpus callosum that we could plausibly regard split-brain patients as two people.

What I would suggest, therefore, is that when you look at the split brain situation from this point of view it does not constitute grounds for the sort of doubt that some philosophers have been raising. Pucchetti, for example, is a well-known Canadian philosopher who has been publishing the suggestion that from the split brain data we can infer that *all* of us are really two conscious individuals in one head, but we happen to be tied together by our corpus callosum. When you cut that out you get evidence that all the time there has been alongside you a mute, and rather stupid, defective individual who is there with some capacity to interfere with your priorities. Given the kind of analysis that I have been offering, that seems to me to go far beyond any evidence that the split brain data provide.

My suggestion would be that we should regard the split brain phenomena as directing more attention to the question: where is the underlying embodiment of the self-supervisory system, especially its higher levels, which I have been giving reasons for regarding as the functional correlate of the unity of our conscious agency? Having said that, let me insist that I do not believe that there is any proof, and I certainly have not offered any, that the possession by an information system of a self-supervisory level is sufficient to constitute, there and then, a centre of conscious awareness. I have given some reasons, I think, for arguing that in somebody who *is* a centre of conscious awareness (someone like ourselves who as a matter of fact – that he or she would be lying to deny – is a centre of conscious experience) the physical correlate which is necessary for our having-conscious-experience is the presence of the self-supervisory level. But it is very much an open question whether the presence of a self-supervisory system could be sufficient. Indeed I shall be advancing some grounds in the next chapter for doubting this, if we allow the self-supervisory concept to be generalized sufficiently to be incorporated in a computer program.

Notes

1 For a fuller account of communication and meaning, see MacKay (1969).

8

Brains and Machines

'Mechanical brains'?

We have been exploring the possibilities of using mechanistic categories to explain the functioning of the brain and this raises a question. Let us just remind ourselves of the essential points. We skeletonized the notion of mechanistic explanation in terms of some flow paths (figure 3.2). We considered the possibilities that in the brain the information from the sensory receptor system is evaluated in a comparison process and, as a result of the evaluation, organizing activity is generated to operate upon an effector system in the field, F, calculated to bring about changes in the field in the direction of the indicated goal-state I_g, which is set by a supervisory or meta-organizing system, one member of a hierarchy that can be expected to extend up through the top left corner of the diagram for as many levels as necessary.

The categories here are mechanistic, albeit in terms of information-flow. That is, we are asking: how does the form of events at one point determine the form of events at another? We are not asking the physicist's question as to where the energy comes from and how it travels. But since it is mechanistic, might it not be possible to build artificial mechanisms which would function in the same sort of way? How much of what interests us in the human brain might also be reproducible in artificial mechanisms?

Machines

Let us begin with a bit of clarification because in this field if we don't distinguish between different meanings of our terms things can get very confused. There are, for a start, several different notions of what we can mean by the term 'machine'. Sometimes it is used, with the adjective 'mere' in front, as a term of dismissal. 'A senseless tool' we mean, when we say a mere machine. That obviously would not be a very worthwhile use of the term for our purpose.

Next we note a respectable use, but one much too vague to be precise: any system that works by push and pull. We use this sort of term to refer, for example, to the mechanistic universe. By this we mean the sort of model of the universe that developed in the early days of science in which the planets – and molecules too – are thought of as interacting by collision or alternatively (as in the Newtonian model) by attraction. Some of the early Greeks, Democritus and the atomists, thought of the molecules as interacting by collision. A system working by push and/or pull is often called 'mechanistic', but this is, in a way, a derivative use of our term and not very germane to our purpose.

A system with a function

A meaning which would be much closer to our purpose is: any system which has a function. What do we mean by a system that has a function? The difference from a system that doesn't goes really quite deep – at least as far as logic goes. If you take the ordinary statements of physics they often take the form: the length of this rod is L. There are two parts to this statement: the rod and its length. You associate the two and you have made a physical statement. But when you say this rod is not long enough to serve as a fishing rod you have invoked its function and introduced a third term: the purpose of catching fish. The logic of talk about function is what Charles Peirce called triadic: it has three terms in the typical statement, rather than the diadic logic of physics. This distinction is non-trivial. It means that your whole perception of a situation which has a function employs a different kind of logic in which every statement has these triple hooks, as it were, to link on to other statements rather than just two. Before you are satisfied with an explanation of what is going on you have to have descriptions in those terms. For example, think of a bridge. A physicist looks at a bridge (*qua* physicist) simply as a structure which has a certain number of parameters that can be specified; there are lengths, strengths and so on. But the functional eye asks whether the bridge is strong enough for the weight of traffic that is going to go over it as lorries get bigger, and so on. Although this may seem a trivial point it actually goes quite deep. And we need to be clear that in passing to thinking of machines as systems with a function we are passing from one kind of logic to another and from one concept of explanation to another.

An artificial agent

Nowadays, when talking about a machine we very often mean an *artificial agent*. When we ask: 'how far can we go to produce in a machine things that would interest us?', we are homing in on the idea of systems with a function, and indeed artificial agents. Now we defined agency as *action under evaluation*. In the case of fishing rods or bridges or whatever, the evaluation is done by us. And when we ask: 'is it strong enough?', it is we who have to evaluate it as strong enough. Similarly in the case of a heater, when we ask: 'is it making the room warm enough?', it is we who evaluate the temperature of the room. But when we introduce something like a thermostat comparator we convert the heater into an artificial agent which embodies a criterion of evaluation. I hope it is clear, and it will certainly be clear by the end of the chapter, that I am not suggesting that there is a little man in there who is doing the evaluating as you or I might do, by deciding that we are too hot or too cold! Nevertheless there is a clear operational sense to saying, in the information engineer's categories, that this particular thing, the box we marked C in our diagrams (figures 3.1 and 3.2), is the evaluator because its function is to adjust the heater in just the way a human being would do if he were doing the evaluating. We have taken one of the knobs that a human being could normally take hold of and we have tied it to part of the mechanism so that the mechanism becomes its own evaluator instead of employing an outside evaluator. This we call an artificial agent.

Comparing the brain with machines

Given this bit of clarification first, let us ask ourselves what we would mean by comparing the brain with machines. Given that we are thinking of machines with a function, artificial agents, there are, I think, three different questions we might have in mind.

1   The first is, how closely does the brain resemble existing mechanisms that we have built for commercial and other purposes? I put this question down really in order to dismiss it as trivial. It is one that is fastened on by many people who want to have a reputation for wisdom and who will say: 'in every age the brain has been compared to the best technology available: first it was compared to clockwork, then to a telephone exchange and nowadays people compare it to computers'. You'll read that in print, but it is nonsense of course; nobody seriously adopts that attitude to the brain. We do not take our models and impose them as Procrustean beds and stretch and squeeze the brain to fit the bed. What we are doing is something quite different. The resemblance to a machine already built for some other purpose is an irrelevance.

2   The second question is a bit more interesting. How far could we go if we wanted to design a machine to imitate the functioning of the brain and body? Here we might find ourselves using (indeed people do) a general purpose digital computer. To this question there is an answer, which at first is exciting and then is rather dull, in the form of a theorem of Turing. But before we go on to that, let us be clear what we mean by a digital computer. In the digital computer the basic process is one of *manipulation of symbols according to rule*. By 'symbols' normally we mean patterns of ones and zeros, electric impulses or things like that. But it is manipulation according to rule in the same sense that a Jacquard weaving loom, for instance, can have the selection of its coloured threads and the sequence in which the weft passes under and over the warp specified according to a rule that is embodied in the pattern of holes punched in a set of cards. It is in that sense that the digital computer can have the selection of the symbolic tokens it manipulates, and the operations it performs on them, specified according to rules embodied in similar patterns – although not usually in punched cards any longer. In modern machines the pattern of symbols and the rules are stored in minute and easily altered blobs of magnetic energy, or sometimes in optical patterns, with huge advantages in the

speed with which they can be pushed around, so that hundreds of millions of operations per second are now commonplace. But the principle of manipulation according to rule is the same in the computer as in an automatic loom or, for that matter, in the distributor of a motor car engine.

Alan Turing, the mathematician, before the Second World War published a famous paper in which he proved, in effect, that any logical performance which you could specify in the form of a finite set of rules could, in principle, be embodied in a machine capable of this kind of general purpose manipulation of symbols. In one sense, he has given a dismissive answer to question 2. There are no limits to the power of an artificial symbol manipulator to imitate the logical pattern of any behaviour that we may care to specify for the machine to tackle, because in a sense you can turn the specification of the tests that you want the machine to meet into a description of a program to guarantee that the machine will meet the tests.

At first this might seem exciting: it seems to promise unlimited scope for the powers of digital symbol processing machines. When you think twice about it, though, it's a bit dull. First of all you don't find it really surprising that if you have set out the procedure for testing whether a machine has a certain logical capacity, then bit by bit you can take the test and say, 'well, I will have to hook up this to that and that to the other and make this do that in this circumstance in order to meet it'.

Secondly, the more you think about it, the more it is clear that the interesting things about human behaviour – inventiveness; falling in love; sensing whether someone is sincere, prejudiced, fair-minded; or making judgements as to whether they are well-informed, generous or wise – all these are things which nobody knows how to specify in the form of a test of whether or not precisely that is present. So the joker in the Turing theorem is not in finding a machine to meet the tests that you might have articulated; the joker is that we don't know how to articulate appropriate rules such that in the presence of a machine meeting those rules we can guarantee that a particular human performance is being perfectly imitated. The process of writing the rules to specify how to imitate a human performance is likely in principle to be an unending process – like the process of describing the physical world. So Turing's theorem doesn't in fact at all guarantee that for any human performance you can always program a machine to imitate it – not even approximately. All it says is: insofar as you understand what you mean by a human performance well enough to break it down into a set of rules, then those rules can be embodied in an appropriate general purpose imitative machine. And of course there are philosophical and psychological grounds for doubting very much whether all human behaviour is reducible to rule-following.

3   There is, however, a third meaning to our concept of comparing the brain with machines. It is expressed by the question: how far can we go in writing rules for the *principles of organization* of human behaviour? This is a question which is sometimes labelled 'theoretical psychology'. Others use the term 'artificial intelligence' (AI) and there are further terms preferred by different people. But what matters is that in our present state of computer science the exciting questions are coming up in terms of question 3. What is aimed at here is not mere external imitation of behaviour but internal imitation or replication of the principles on which human behaviour is organized.

Now this question makes it much clearer that we are on to an empirical science which can only proceed, like physics or any other, by trying to build hypothetical templates. Hold them up against reality and see how far they match; and then improve them progressively by further trial-and-error and experiment. There is no question of a Turing's theorem saying that we can guarantee that this can be done without limit. We just have to get on with it and see how well it goes. In the process, as the label 'theoretical psychology' suggests, it may be that our understanding of the functioning of the brain may advance just as much as our ability to provide good imitations. Typical questions, you see, would be: how can we design an artificial processor which can derive an internal description of a world of three-dimensional objects given only a few two-dimensional pictures from a television camera, or, conversely, how can we persuade it to build a three-dimensional model accurately given only some verbal descriptions? Or how well can we write rules for the giving of intelligent expert advice? And can we design a computer system such that, if it is provided with a lot of samples of an expert's giving his advice in answer to particular questions, it can induce (develop, that is, symbolic representations of) the principles on which the expert is giving his advice, so that it in turn can give answers to similar questions and can answer further questions of the kind why did you say this, or on what grounds did you choose that as the answer?

All of these things may sound science fiction to us, but they are not;

they are reality. They are commercial reality and there are centres of such activity in many cities where I think a lot of money is being made right now by answering questions of that sort. With this kind of sample and this kind of clarification of the sort of questions we are asking, I am going to take it for granted for the sake of our discussion that there is nothing unrealistic in imagining a rule-driven generator of intelligent human behaviour which, after enough generations of activity, becomes indistinguishable in most respects from the behaviour you would expect of a human being. We are talking, of course, about information-handling behaviour. We are not talking about the ability to jump a certain number of feet in the air (though that might or might not be a trivial extension); we are talking about the things that interest us about the brain in relation to what we call mental activity. I am going to be asking for the rest of this chapter: what if we were at not merely the 'fifth generation' of computers, as they call it today, but the umpteenth generation in which there were no noticeable differences between most of the behaviour, in a suitable dialogue situation, of the artificially generating system and that of a human being. I see no particular difficulty in imagining, at least in a century or two, a domain in which conversation with artificial inter-locutors and reliance on their judgement and so forth could occupy a lot of human activity.

At this point we could spend much time thinking about which aspects of the mechanical agent's performance might still be left over that we could not yet be satisfied with as human. But the questions I want to move on to are, I think, in some ways much more interesting.

Is there anyone there?

The first of these questions is quite fundamental. Suppose we do have in front of us this artificial agent giving all the signs that a human being would give of intelligent capability of handling information and responding to dialogue. Is there anyone there? I want to stick to that way of putting the question for the moment because I think it gets to the roots of our common sense better than some other forms. Is there anyone there, given that there is an entity in front of you and that from that entity there will come conversational exchange? It doesn't have to come by way of a typewriter of course; already we have got rather guttural artificial talkers. So you have all the possibilities of interacting as you would with a conscious human agent; but *is* there anyone there?

Now some people would argue that if the rules have been sufficiently carefully and cleverly designed you will not be able to tell the difference. In fact Turing himself was inclined to talk this way. On those grounds many people imagine that there are philosophical reasons for saying that there *must* be somebody there because you can't tell the difference. But this, of course, if you think of yourself as the individual in question, is clearly nonsense. There is all the difference in the world between whether you are in fact there as a conscious agent and whether what is sitting there is your body but you happen to be, for clinical or other reasons, unconscious.

Furthermore, there is a very simple *Gedanken experiment* which we can treat ourselves to which shows there is no rational basis for the answer being yes. Suppose you go to the theatre and you watch Joe Bloggs, the actor, playing Hamlet in the famous soliloquy. Joe does a good job: before you, in a certain poetic, artistic sense, there clearly is Hamlet agonizing over his decision. You follow the twists and turns of this thought; you enter into his mind. But if I were to ask you: 'how many *conscious centres of awareness* are there on the stage?', surely your answer would be, just one. There is only Joe Bloggs there. Joe is imitating Hamlet quite well, but Hamlet is not there in addition.

Now how would it sound if the producer, having heard you say this, were to say 'give me a little bit longer; I haven't had long enough to program Joe to be a really good imitation of Hamlet; but give me another generation or two and we will have a Joe who will imitate Hamlet, who will generate Hamlet's behaviour on the same principles as Hamlet, sufficiently that you won't be able to tell the difference'. What would your answer be? It wouldn't make a hoot of difference: no amount of perfection in the imitation of Hamlet by Joe will bring Hamlet into being as a conscious centre of awareness in addition to Joe. There would still be only one person there and that is Joe. Hamlet's behaviour is there, but Hamlet is not – at least I can think of no non-superstitious reason for supposing that he is. My argument then is a very simple one: *a fortiori* if, instead of Joe Bloggs the actor, you put on the stage an IBM computer suitably programmed to imitate not merely Hamlet's external behaviour but also the principles of his behaviour, it would be even less rational to conclude from the perfection of the imitation that Hamlet is now present. There is no rational path at all from the progressive improvement of an imitation of the behaviour of X to the conclusion that X, as a conscious agent, is there present. There is nobody there; only an IBM computer doing its stuff. Or there is nobody extra there; only Joe Bloggs doing a very good imitation of somebody who isn't there.

My first point, then, is that no matter how much perfection we expect in the principles of organization of behaviour in artificial intelligence, there are – contrary to what many AI protagonists have claimed in print – no rational grounds whatever for supposing that there is *anybody there*, for supposing that there is a conscious centre of awareness, aware of us as we are aware of what is going on in front of us.

Can a computer understand?

Now there is a second question, and it is important to see that it is not the same question: can a computer, suitably embellished on the lines we have imagined, be said to *understand*? Can it be said to understand what is said to it, for example. Here it is important to realize that in talking about 'a computer' we are giving ourselves an underspecified state description, we are drawing a mental curtain around a lot of stuff that is going on that we don't want to know about. We just want to see what results on the far side of the curtain. It is like the organs in church: you normally conceal the rather ugly bellows that are flapping up and down as the organist is running his fingers over the keys. But let's take the curtains off. Let's look inside. What is happening is the continual consultation of sets of rules for symbol manipulation. And when you think about it, the same principle – however elaborate – that we have imagined in our mechanism could also be implemented by using, let us say, a human slave to consult a printed book of rules and do all the necessary fetching, exchanging and delivering of symbolic tokens according to those rules. He would be slow, of course, but never mind that; we are not in the business of supposing that the presence or absence of understanding or of conscious experience depends on how quickly the organism operates.

So, as we often used to point out in the early days of computing back in the 1940s and 1950s, such a slave need have no comprehension of the meaning of the calculating or other process he is helping to instantiate. It could be his master's tax bill or the number of legions needed to invade Britain but he need never know or understand – he doesn't even need to understand the processes of addition and subtraction; he simply has to place tokens in positions appropriate to his orders. Conversely, if the slave were replaced by an automatic look-up mechanism with equivalent functions of the sort that we have been presupposing so far, it would be quite baseless to credit that mechanism or system with any more understanding of the process of calculation than the slave had. If a slave can do it without understanding, then a machine can do it without understanding, and the fact that the system works as if there were somebody there, understanding what you said to it, doesn't in the least have a tendency logically or rationally to imply that inside the box behind the curtain there is somebody who is understanding, or indeed that any understanding is going on.

Now J. R. Searle, in his 1984 Reith lectures, has innocently recapitulated many of the arguments on this topic that circulated in the 1950s, but I think I should point out one or two points of divergence between what he had to say and what I want to argue, in case the two get confused. In the first place he confuses the issue at this point by claiming that 'in the human sense computers do not follow rules at all ... they only act in accord with formal procedures'. Well, I regard that as a distinction without a significant difference: we all know what we mean by Jacquard looms being rule-guided systems and that is something which does not affect the point at issue here. Although – as you will already realize – I agree with Searle that digital computers do not *think*, I doubt whether he has found the best way to express the distinction that we need, because the sense in which an automatic loom follows rules is close enough to the human for a human operator to take the place of the automatic card reader and follow the same rules.

What Searle should have said, I think, is that in a psychological or mentalistic sense computers don't follow rules or, better perhaps, that the conscious mental process which we call *understanding the meaning of a rule and obeying it* is not embodied in the rule-following processes of a digital computer any more than it is in those of a Jacquard loom or a motor engine. If we replace the automatic manipulative machinery of the computer by a human slave as I was suggesting earlier – a slave required to consult a book of rules – then of course we do have a mental process going on in the slave of rule-following. But as we saw, this is irrelevant to the *meaning* of the computing operations, which the slave need not understand as such. All he needs to know is where to go to pick up a token and where to dump it again, according to the rules in the book. The slave may be mentally busy thinking and acting according to the meaning of the rules in his book, but there is nobody there thinking – working out mentally – what the calculation means.

Searle makes a similar point using the example of a room in which a non-Chinese speaker successfully follows rules for the manipulation and exchange of Chinese symbols, so that Chinese speakers can engage in meaningful communication with the system he operates although he himself understands no Chinese. He may act as if he understands, but the appearance is deceptive. And Searle argues, on similar lines to these earlier arguments, that if the manipulative functions of the non-Chinese speaker were successfully taken over by a digital computer there would be no rational grounds for claiming that the computer understood Chinese.

So far, on this point, there is no disagreement with Searle, but then he goes on, in my view at least, to spoil it all by saying, 'only brains can understand'. Here he has crossed the line between what we have been calling the I-story category and the brain-story category. The conclusion that is appropriate here in these terms is that only people can understand, or at any rate, only *agents* can understand. Understanding is not something that it makes sense to predicate of brains: it is not brains but people who think, understand and have other events of conscious experience to bear witness to. So insofar as the word 'understand' is taken to be one of the terms in the language of conscious experience, it would be inept to say that 'brains understand' for the same reason that it is inept to say that 'machines understand'. Neither brains nor machines understand. That is not what they are categorically equipped to do.

Understanding by artificial agents?

This does not, however, answer the question which, I believe, is of interest to us and which I think perhaps Searle dismisses too quickly by this move of his. The question is not whether a *computer* can understand, because a computer is, as we have been discussing it, a symbol manipulator pure and simple, replaceable by a lot of morons who only know how to follow rules that have nothing to do with the meaning of what the computer is doing. The question that does interest us is whether there is any sense in which an *artefact*, that is to say an artificial and mechanistic system (which almost certainly will embody such a computer), can be said to understand.

You may be surprised to find that I want to argue that there *is* such a sense. And it is for a very simple practical reason: that in an all too meaningful sense it is possible even today to build artificial mechanical agents that can *mis*understand.

Misunderstanding by artificial agents

Let me sketch what I mean. Here is a motor car assembly line. Along the bench higgledy-piggledy there are human agents for assembling things and robots for assembling things and both of them are acoustically controlled, that is to say the foreman shouts orders at certain times. The robots are equipped with artificial ears and with speech recognizing machinery (it all exists). At an appropriate moment the foreman shouts 'Wait!', because something has gone wrong and the line has to stop. And one of the robots lifts the object it is holding and puts it on a weighing machine. Now what is the obvious way of describing this if not to say that the robot 'misunderstood'. All the other operators including robots understood, but this one misunderstood. I put it to you that it would be carrying philosophical nicety to perverse lengths to deny that this is a proper use of the word 'misunderstand'. The robot is being perceived by you in functional terms as an agent, as an evaluative agent, as a goal-directed agent, but an agent whose superordinate goals (top priorities) are at least influenceable by the foreman. The foreman does his stuff towards the robot as he would towards a human. The rest of them, both humans and robots, understand (why shouldn't we say understand?) correctly. Certainly one of them gives clear behavioural evidence of misunderstanding.

If it is possible in that sense, and I agree it is not the fullest sense of the word 'understand', but in that important sense for an artificial agent to misunderstand, it seems to me it would be perversely restrictive to deny the concept of understanding. But notice the cost. We now must distinguish between the concept of understanding and the concept of having a conscious experience to bear witness to – because this kind of understanding is behaviouristic understanding. It is a shorthand term, and a useful one, to describe a category of behaviour. To misunderstand is to have a conditional readiness to behave in a manner not matched to the selective function (the meaning) of the communication that was sent. The misunderstanding of the communication to the robot is betokened not by the fact that symbols have been pushed around inside (that is nothing to do with the understanding), but by the fact that the state of conditional readiness is mismatched to that which the communication meant. The communication has not evoked its intended meaning, its intended selective function, on the state of conditional readiness for action by the robot. The robot, then, is an artificial agent which I am suggesting we ought to credit with understanding without crediting it with conscious experience. There is no need to do that; indeed there are lots of grounds for scepticism there. But 'misunderstanding', it seems to me, is a useful category in the context where dialogue with a robot is possible.

A fresh lease of life for behaviourism

We thus arrive at a realization that dialogue may be possible in the absence of conscious experience. We need to recognize the meaningfulness of agency which includes the capacity to understand and misunderstand communications without presupposing that the agent is conscious. We can have unconscious agency which has in this sense a behaviouristic psychology. It seems to me indeed that much of the early behaviouristic psychology could usefully be resurrected for some of these purposes on condition that we include in the term 'behaviour' the *internal* behaviour of the supervisory levels of agency – the making of internal models, resetting of priorities and so forth. All these activities that we are supposing could be mechanically engineered must be included in the whole category of the behaviour of the artificial agent. You see then that there is all the difference in the world between talking of a computer understanding, which is nonsense (I agree with Searle), and talking of an artificial agent understanding, which in this sense is valid.

Now you may ask why psychologists junked behaviouristic psychology, by and large. The answer I think is generally recognized to be that behaviouristic psychology was wrong in what somebody has called 'feigning unconsciousness'. It is almost charming to read in Watson and the early founders of behaviourism the prudish way in which they pretended that their subjects – and by implication they themselves, I suppose – were not conscious agents. Consciousness was a dirty word; one kept it out because behaviour was all one could measure. They were infatuated with the observer relationship in physics and doing their best to replicate it. What I am suggesting is that although it made that kind of psychology progressively worthless for the study of human behaviour in its more interesting manifestations, it does not necessarily invalidate it as a discipline for the classification and anatomizing of the behaviour of artificial agents.

The unpredictability of artificial agents in dialogue

As I have already pointed out, dialogue with artificial agents is now a practical possibility. In dialogue with even an artificial agent the underspecification, the indeterminacy that I pointed to in the last chapter, would apply: the reciprocal relation between two agents in dialogue makes each indeterminate to the other. There is no reason technically why it should not apply to the artificial agent that we are now talking about. So that in your interaction with a (suitably equipped) artificial agent you would sense, as you would with a human agent, that indeterminacy in the other as a reflection of your own indeterminacy to yourself.

Consciousness in artificial agents?

In case anyone thinks that the remaining issue of consciousness or unconsciousness is a trivial one, let me remind you that it was Augustine, long before Descartes, who pointed out that you have only to doubt your own consciousness to have established it. The idea that it is a non-issue has long been recognized as nonsense.

As to attributing consciousness to others, if anyone were to try the old line that 'if one hasn't got a suitable test, then it is a "meaningless" question whether a particular organism is conscious or not', I hold that they would be going beyond what is philosophically justified. It is, you see, a matter of fact whether or not you or I or any other organism is conscious. Let us turn it upon you[1] as you sit there: let us imagine that all of the rest of us consider the organism in that chair (you), and having entered into conclave, come to the conclusion that although it is a convincing imitation, there is nobody there. There would be one individual, I put it to you, who would know we are wrong on a matter of fact, and that would be you. So consciousness does not hang on framing a suitable test. It is a question of fact. It is an ontological question.

Somebody may ask what I mean by 'consciousness'; is it the ability to tell an I-story? It is certainly not the *ability* to tell an I-story, because somebody who had lost the power of speech could still be conscious. What I said in the first chapter is that there are two sources of data. The prime source we conventionally call the 'data of conscious experience' and to these inner, first person, experiences we bear witness as best we can in the I-story. So the prime question is not can I *tell* an I-story, but are there data that *demand* an I-story, however incompetent I may be to frame an I-story to do justice to the data? As to the further question of consciousness in animals, I would feel it irrational to deny that most animals have conscious experience – I don't know how far down. Certainly any animal with a supervisory level would seem to me to have a *prima facie* case for being credited with conscious experience. Pain, for example, would seem to me to be a meaningful category, rather than 'pain-like behaviour' as the more absurd behaviourists used to say. [*The question of consciousness in artificial agents is taken up again towards the end of the present chapter.*]

Rule-followers: the end of the road?

With all we have been envisaging here, we have been considering the workings of a system that is a rule-follower. But the following of rules is, in an important sense, not a very exciting source of fundamental novelty. That's the first objection to the idea that in a rule-following imitator of principles of organization we can have reached the end of the road.

There is another limitation for rule-followers that ought to be mentioned. This was spelt out by Karl Popper in 1950, for a reason similar to the one that we have been discussing in relation to logical relativity, but he made a different point from it. He pointed out that any rule-following computer is bound to be limited in its capacity to calculate the future of a universe that includes itself, because in order to complete its rule-operated calculations it would need to have information as to the outcome of its calculations (in order to feed them into the equations which would predict its *own* future). Thus it would always be chasing its own tail, short of data for its calculations.

Now this incapacity of a computer to predict its own future must be distinguished from the point that I was making in relation to logical relativity, which was that regardless of your interest in, or capability of, predicting your own future there *does not exist* a specification of the immediate future of your state of conditional readiness which could logically claim to be beliefworthy by you. This is quite a different point – a logical point. (Popper's is a cognate point – that a predicting machine, however perfect as a calculator, cannot in principle predict its own future.)

So we come back to our question: is this the end of the line – is what I have been discussing so far all that we can hope for from mechanistic systems by way of replication of the features in human beings that interest us?

Internal experimentation: what analogue processes have to offer

Now this is a question that I found myself up against in the late 1940s and I came up with an answer then that I would like to sketch briefly as an indication of a whole further class of possibilities that, I think, might be of interest. It involves us, I'm afraid, in one or two more basic distinctions. The first of these is between the whole class of machine whose selective operation is performed according to rule (a digital computer being the standard exemplar) and a class of machine or mechanism whose selective operations are performed as a result of an internal experiment.

What I mean by this is illustrated by two ways of adding two and three. One possibility is to count two pebbles into a jar and then to drop another three pebbles in and then to count the result. That would be 'digital' calculation of 2 plus 3 and the answer would be 5 as a result of the process of counting. Another would be to perform a physical experiment: take a graduated measuring jar, pour 2 cm^3 of water in; pour 3 cm^3 of water in; measure the result: 5 cm^3. That's a physical experiment. That is an appeal to nature: let nature perform what nature does according to nature's laws and I will read off the answer and interpret it as a substitute for what I would otherwise have had to do by thinking or counting. It is called analogue computing and this process is, of course, a totally different conception from that of manipulating symbols according to rule. Appealing to nature, letting nature give you the answer (provided that you have suitably constrained the conditions) is quite a different operation.

Let me show you a nice illustration of a mechanism on the analogue principle, designed in the last century by Sir William Thomson (later Lord Kelvin) for calculating tidal heights in India (plate 21). It is a great hunk of hardware – cranks, pulley wheels and cord. Why do we call it a 'calculator'? Only, of course, because we are prepared to attribute to the movements of the various pens and so on the significance of the sums of various sinusoidal components of tidal motion: the final movement of the pen on the drum represents the tides on that assumption alone. To suppose that there was any rational ground for calling such a thing a 'thinking machine', or that there is somebody there thinking about tides, would be sheer animistic superstition – just as with a digital machine – but it does illustrate the principle of making a physical experiment in order to get the answer to our uncertainty. Instead of carrying out a logical process according to logical rules, this is now a physical process according to physical rules.

[*Analogue methods have the merit that adjacent states in the calculator correspond to adjacent situations in the solution. They can also economically admit of simultaneous parallel calculation across a wide front. The effects of small changes and of gradual trends can therefore be explored; integration performed; minima and stable states discovered; knife edges and bifurcations represented – all with a rapidity and naturalness not possible with a digital computer.*]

'Intelligent' machinery is characterized by the presence of branch-points in the course of events at which one out of several possibilities must be selected, the outcome being determined, at least in part, by what amounts to a physical experiment. True, one could always 'in principle' approximate to a continuous transition as closely as desired using a digital computer if one could afford enough digits; but even this costly strategy could not be expected always to insure against unforeseen blindspots or anomalies in the resulting process. For example, however finely one approximates to a 45 degree inclined plane by a series of steps, their surface area is always $\sqrt{2}$ times too big!

Any light-hearted rejection, however, of one technique in favour of the other would seem to be unjustified. For many problems in mathematics and mathematical logic, the characteristics of digital computers make them particularly attractive. Where high numerical accuracy is essential, they are much more economical. But if long term retentivity is naturally a digital function, the conservation of short term equilibrium is equally naturally an analogue one.

In digital mechanisms, a quantal process ensures precision, and order and structure are primary concepts; magnitude continuity and trend are derivative. In analogue mechanisms magnitude, continuity and trend are primary concepts; order and structure are abstractions.

The marriage of analogue and digital strengths: continuous variation of the probabilities of discontinuous events

The question which interested me, and which I tackled back in the 1940s and 1950s, was: what qualitatively new possibilities open up if we think of a mechanism that could combine these two principles – the digital and the analogue? The most logically natural way of combining the two principles, once one thinks it through, is to allow the physical experimentation aspect of what is going on to control or modulate the *probabilities* of events which would otherwise function according to a precise rule.

[*'Once one thinks it through' in the sentence above refers principally to thinking about the kind of thing information is – information, of course, being what the brain or automaton is to handle, store and make use of. Information is that which justifies a representation. If we want to think about the information gathered up into a representation (for example, into the image on a photographic plate) we are interested not only in its geographical structure – the optically independent areas of the photographic plate – but also in the reliance we can place on the density of the image at each point – how closely it does justice to what was photographed. Two aerial photographs, for example, may happen to have the same grey level in a certain area, but in the one, thanks to superior film and camera and atmospheric conditions, the grey levels may be much more tightly tied to the intensity of the object photographed than in the other. It therefore is more informative. If we want to measure how much more reliance we should place on the evidence from the one representational pattern than from the other in this respect – how much more weight we should give to it – the units are those of* metrical *information content (normally a function of the inverse of the variance).*

It was as a result of this 'thinking through' in about 1948 that] I became very excited about extending the conceptual and information processing range of automata by equipping them to take account of the *weight and relevance of information as well as its logical structure.* The primary requirement here is that the weight attached to evidence should be represented by a separate physical variable which can determine the contribution it makes to the pattern of action in given circumstances. It seemed natural to regard the all-or-none precision of the digital computer as a special and limiting case of a more general non-discrete kind of information-processing, much as the integers are special cases in the continuum of real numbers (from MacKay, 1949).

The control of transition probabilities

A simple illustration

Think, as an example, of a gun which has an uncertain trigger, and suppose that we have attached to the trigger a number of springs in different directions and we vary the tension on those springs (figure 8.1). That is a typical analogue operation. It is a typical physical experiment: combination of 'weights' either positively or negatively takes place on an 'analogue' principle to determine the probability of action of the gun. There is going to be some point at which the combination of tensions will be just right to pull the trigger back far enough to fire the gun – indeed there will be several combinations. The firing of the gun is a discrete event: it is like the firing of an element in a digital computer, a one or a zero; but its probability is modified according to the tensions of the springs.

You could call these springs physical representations of *conditional probabilities.* Let us see how the word 'conditional' would come in. The tensions depend upon the positions of a number of pegs, P_1, P_2, etc., to which springs from the trigger are attached. But suppose now that the position of each peg (to which springs from several guns are attached) is shifted sideways according to the amount of firing that other, similarly arranged, guns have been doing. The whole resultant set-up would then show the conditional probability that if gun A fires, that

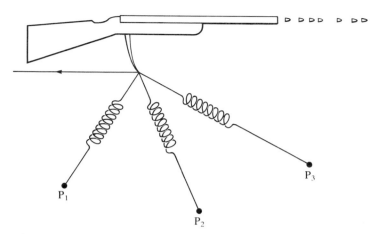

Figure 8.1   A simple illustration of analogue control of a discrete process.

will change the probability that gun B will fire, and so on. You can have a hierarchy of probability that if this happens, but not that, then this will happen, provided that something else hasn't – to as many terms as you like.

In case this sounds extravagant, let us remind ourselves that in thinking about the nervous system we saw that the typical nerve cell can exist in a range of possible states according to its 'bias', from 'spontaneously active' at one extreme to 'heavily suppressed' at the other. The cell's probability of 'firing' (or being activated) depends not only on its metabolic state but also on the precise relative timing and layout of hundreds or even thousands of incoming signals. Inhibitory or excitatory signals from other cells, or chemical signals from the bloodstream, can vary the cell's individual 'conditional readiness' so as to modulate continuously its probability of firing, or its frequency of firing, in given circumstances. This control of transition probability is just what an information engineer would need in order to make a flexible system in which weight-of-evidence would play the rational part we want it to (this paragraph from MacKay, 1951).

We have in the nervous system networks of neurons where there could be thousands of connections whose points of contact with cells were adjustable. Their interrelationships are adjustable precisely in the way that that sort of crude spring model illustrates. The strength of the connection varies the probability that if one nerve cell fires in the presence of a certain activity in another cell, but not in the presence of something else which is inhibitory, then a particular cell will give out an impulse. Moreover, repercussions of the impulse will come back round and have a feedback effect on some of the others.

Turning to man-made systems, we have already seen in figure 2.7 an example of an artificial associative net, again using dozens or hundreds of connections, where the probabilities of operation depend on how many signals are coming in and in what particular pattern. The weights, the couplings, are automatically adjusted by the associative mechanism so as to provide the equivalent of learning. The details don't matter, but this highly promising class of network for carrying out things like recognizing speech sounds, faces or signatures works in just the kind of way that we found in the late 1940s and early 1950s was attractive in opening up scope for something different from rule-guided behaviour. Making physical experiments, or if you like allowing nature and physical laws to play a part complementary to the logical laws and rules embodied in programs, gives you a much more flexible and exciting category of artificial mechanism.

Intelligent behaviour

The question is, of course, how we would envisage this as generating intelligent behaviour. When we speak of a man of intellect we have in mind something which quite transcends the man's ability to calculate and to make deductions. He must indeed be able to follow and test and carry through trains of reasoning, and to store information and instructions. But when we admire his intellect it is not for these abilities alone; it is rather for judgement, the ability to weigh evidence, a sense of proportion, ingenuity, initiative and originality shown in their exercise. It is in this reflective activity that the features which distinguish intellect from mere information-processing ability emerge most prominently. The point I want to stress is that some of the most distinctive of these features concern the metrical aspect of information, which is specially suited to representation by continuous variables. For example a man of intellect can:

take cognizance of the weight as well as the structure of evidence;

take tentative steps not logically forced, yet rationally disciplined, by his data, setting his threshold of significance neither too high nor too low;

limit the complexity of his exploratory repertoire to match the skill he has acquired so far in using it, so that the information per trial is optimized;

steer his intellectual explorations by a sense of the proximity of a solution (the ability to tell when he is 'getting warmer');

generate a *limited* range of *promising* hypotheses or possible conclusions compatible with the data;

perceive analogies spontaneously.

How well can the sort of stochastic system we are thinking of meet the challenge represented by such features? The key feature required, which is offered by neural mechanisms, and illustrated by our guns and springs, is transition-probability control.

Weight of evidence and the threshold of evidence

What I pointed out in those early papers on mind-like behaviour in artefacts was that we have two important parameters – variables – to lay hold on and determine.

The obvious form of variable to represent the 'weight' of evidence would be the strength of the signal embodying the evidence, in terms either of the amplitude or of the number of signal elements recruited in parallel.

Secondly, the mechanization of intellect requires facilities for evaluating the *sufficiency of evidence*. In real life no finite body of evidence, for however long we accumulate it, can *prove* a generalization. We must constantly draw essential conclusions from insufficient data, while recognizing that the correct conclusion may have escaped us among an infinity of alternatives. A continuous range of attitudes is therefore possible between the precipitate confidence of the scatter-brain whose decisions are too frequent and ill-considered and the impotent caution of the fastidious logician. They differ in what we might call the *threshold of evidence* below which no conclusion is reached. I can illustrate these variables by two ratios in the case of our guns and springs.

1   The ratio of signal to bias, S/B. The first ratio that is going to be important is the ratio of input signal to bias, S/B. A very weak pull on the spring is not going to make much happen if the bias against firing

is very large, but if the bias is very small the same weak pull will have a large effect on the probability.

2   The ratio of bias to noise, B/N. The second can be thought of by imagining that this whole system of guns and springs is vibrating. (In the real world of nerve cells and tiny objects the vibrations are thermal vibrations at least and the cell has natural fluctuations in excitability.) There is always what is called 'noise' in the system so there is nothing unrealistic in introducing this in a model of intelligent behaviour; in fact we need it. We have then a system which is vibrating and therefore, even if you held everything still, there would be some tiny probability that the gun might fire. This would depend upon how far the trigger was already pulled back. As the trigger is pulled there will come a point at which the vibration will certainly fire it. (Another possible source of 'noise' would be that the signals coming in to pull the triggers might also be vibrating, and their 'noise' of variation would provide another statistical source of uncertainty as to how the whole thing will function. Formally, however, all the above may be attributed to the existence of the random component, N, in the input. The probability of an 'incorrect' firing of a gun will be an increasing function of the ratio N/B.)

So we have here a system which, in addition to any logical interrelations dictated by the positions of the springs, guns and triggers, has these two variables, one of them representing, as it were, how strong the tugs or pulls are which determine the probability that the gun will fire and the other, B/N, how reluctant the guns are to fire. These two provide different classes of behaviour which range from the totally chaotic at one end to the digital precision extreme at the other. If the noise vanishes and everything operates on a strength which is large compared with the bias, we are back with an ordinary digital machine. (I have, in fact, found it more helpful, especially when thinking of possible brain models, to talk of the disciplining of potentially random activity, rather than the perturbation of potentially digital precision.) This then is a general-purpose symbol-manipulating system which also embodies the notion of a probability matrix.

[*The paper from 1949 spells out in more detail the types of behaviour which will result, in an 'intelligent' machine, from the four basic combinations of these parameters. The last is the most interesting.*] The terms used are those applicable to analogous manifestations in human beings, and are of course purely metaphorical. In human beings the terms connote much more.

1 If S/B and N/B are both low, words such as dull, sluggish, moronic, forgetful, lazy or unreliable can be given behaviouristic significance in relation to the machine.

2 If S/B is still low, and N/B is increased, characteristics analogous to imbecility appear. Logical sequences are short and disjointed, stored information becomes distorted and hallucinatory impressions arise, motor activity is aimless, and so on. These conditions can of course be present in varying degrees.

3 If N/B is low, and S/B is increased, behaviour becomes more normal, typical features being reliability, lack of imagination, promptness of response, and so forth.

4 If S/B is high, and N/B is increased at suitable points, the frequency of 'bright ideas' will tend to increase, each being normally followed-up in a logical fashion. If N/B increases further, however, the frequency of new ideas may reach a level at which normal functioning is impaired. In a sense then we have an illustration of the familiar aphorism that 'genius is next door to insanity'; but the 'insanity' of this extreme case where N/B and S/B are both high (in the various forms which will differ according to the location of the noise) will be quite different in character from the 'imbecility' of group 2 (from MacKay, 1949).

It might be biologically advantageous for a brain built of such elements to have ways of adjusting the overall levels, particularly of N/B, according to the task in hand.

Exploratory activity

In all exploratory activity, the ability to sense *gradients* is vital. To this end, an information engineer would use the principle of 'replication with variation'. This means that instead of using a single representation of a situation as a basis for internal experimental trials, he would run several near-replicas in parallel, each different in some parameter from the others. The difference between simultaneous neighbouring outcomes could then generate an error vector which would greatly increase the speed of convergence of the exploratory process. There is already some evidence, mainly from sensory systems, that the neural population lends itself to multiple parallel processing on these lines.

This is closely related to the question above as to how new hypotheses can be generated spontaneously with a better than average chance of success. With a digital code, the method of random perturbation, which so amused Gulliver in Laputa, fails because there is near-zero probability that physically neighbouring states of digital code symbols will represent conceptually neighbouring possibilities. In a system in which states of affairs are represented by states of conditional readiness to reckon with them, however, physically neighbouring states can in general represent conceptually neighbouring states of affairs. Small perturbations in such a physical representation will generally make small changes in its representational significance. This means incidentally that such representations are much less dangerously vulnerable to noise than groups of arbitrary code symbols. More to the point, it means that small experimental modifications have a relatively low probability of making transitions to wildly irrelevant hypotheses; moreover, the spontaneous transitions that do take place are automatically under the constraints of the data embodied in the current representation.

A human thinker can of course be wrong in thinking himself near the best solution. He may have reached only a small local dip in a plateau, rather than the valley bottom he seeks. If our mechanized system is to avoid such traps, it must try a range of variations on a small scale with high discrimination, and others on a larger scale with lower discrimination to sense more general trends. It may well be that the familiar benefits of practice in problem solving arise partly from its influence on the range-distribution explored by our own brain mechanism.

What of the ability to perceive analogies spontaneously? Bear in mind that we envisage each situation perceived as represented internally by a combination of subroutines which bring the organizing system into a matching state of conditional readiness for that situation. If situations find themselves satisfactorily matched by combinations having one or more subroutines in common, this means that from the agent's standpoint they *are* analogous in the respect represented by the shared subroutine. A system on this principle, then, needs no special additional machinery to enable it to spot analogies. This will happen automatically, provided that the internal situation-descriptors used by the supervisory system are the component subroutines engaged in matching the situation perceived (from MacKay, 1956). [*(The preceding four paragraphs are drawn from MacKay, 1949, 1956, 1959, 1984b.)*]

To sum up briefly on this, when you combine all these possibilities – and some of them are being very actively pursued now in the study of 'Boltzmann machines' (Boltzmann being the physicist who developed the theory of 'noise') – it turns out that machines of this sort with variable noise levels can, as it were, let their hair down with a high noise level for a time and make a lot of explorations to match the input. Then you can turn the noise down again and the networks 'anneal' themselves in a new mode of organization which matches the new input (Ackley et al., 1985). Such Boltzmann machinery has a very exciting future both as technology and as a model of some brain processes.

Cooperativity within a machine

Let me also point out that, as you can guess from this, variation of the average bias B (or the ratio B/S) could have another important function in relation to exploratory activity. If you have got thousands of elements interconnected along these lines, whether you think of springs or electrical connections or whatever, there are going to be modes of cooperativity which are *qualitatively* new in the sense in which a flame is a qualitatively new phenomenon when you ignite gas and air mixed in a burner. As long as things are un-ignited they don't cooperate in the self-exciting way which gives rise to the new entity, a flame.

The entities to treat are not the electrical or physical elements but patterns or waves of their activity, with laws of motion and interaction of their own, relatively free to move through the substrate as ripples can move over the surface of a pool, or waves of excitement through a crowd.

As in the nervous system, so also in the artificial devices of the above sort, we have to expect qualitatively new possibilities along the lines of cooperativity. In a stochastic system whose elements are anatomically rich in couplings to neighbours, the effective number of degrees of freedom (the number of effectively independent controls) depends directly on the strength of those couplings. With a low enough bias, cooperativity will set in so that large domains will switch state simultaneously, and the repertoire of the system will have relatively few independent modes. As the average bias B is raised, the average size of cooperative domains will be reduced, increasing the effective number of degrees of freedom and hence the potential richness of the repertoire. It is easy to see how this mechanism could be used during development (whether physical or intellectual) to allow the complexity of a repertoire to grow in step with the complexity of the subroutines evolved to represent (by matching) the world it has to deal with (from MacKay, 1956, 1984b).

You can see that my best hopes for the production of really human-like intelligent agency, including the internal self-supervisory agency that we have talked about as the correlate of mental activity, are pinned on mechanisms that rely on appropriate combinations of rule-following on the one hand and internal experimentation of this string-tugging sort on the other.

Consciousness: the possible importance of construction by growth

Suppose that we succeed in this beyond our wildest dreams. Once more let me ask: would we have any rational grounds for saying there is someone there *now* – that now, at last, we have brought into being an artificially conscious agent?

I'm afraid my answer would have to be: no, because there is a difference still between all we have been talking about and the brain, and I think it may not be a trivial one, although at this point I am out at the frontier of my ignorance. In all these artificial devices the material world serves under constraints, which you might call 'cutting across the grain'. We build these things out of hunks of matter which *we* shape. If they are made of wood there are grain marks, if they are made of metal they are cut, sawn and cast rather than *grown*. I suspect there may be a whole world of difference in a scientific sense between the sort of conditional probability matrix that can 'grow' in a system of that sort and the sort that can grow in a system like the brain, where the elementary parts develop their shape by growth – that is to say, by the following through of the fundamental principles of physics and chemistry right from the quarks upward. For that reason I think we must maintain reasonable scepticism as to whether the embellishments of introducing these new principles would give us any more grounds for believing that we have in front of us as a result somebody who has an I-story to tell as we have.

In the late 1940s I wondered whether we could go so far and said: 'Suppose we jump the gap which is deductively unbridgeable and conclude that what we now have is a conscious agent'. I have given reasons above for questioning whether we are entitled to jump it. I think it really does matter that we distinguish between saying two possible things. The first is: I can see no difference between the behaviour of a human being and the behaviour of this other (the man-made) object. The second is: I have the same grounds therefore for crediting this other object with conscious experience. The reason we credit each other with consciousness is, in part, that we know that there exists one sample, namely ourselves, in which having a particular kind of structure and ancestry *does* go with consciousness. So it would be irrational of me, I think, when short of other evidence, to deny *you* conscious experience. But in the case of our artefact I think the boot is on the other foot. It would be irrational of me to have too low a threshold for crediting the artefact with conscious experience, given that the artefact is one of a series which has, as far as I can see, continuity of development from the thermostat.

I am distinguishing, in other words, between the two great classes of mechanism known to us, the artificial mechanism whose structure is imposed by us, and the natural mechanism – the biological mechanism – whose structure is grown. I think there is a legitimate doubt as to whether what makes us have conscious experience may not have something non-accidental related to the detailed biophysics of our embodiment. If we ask whether it matters what brains are made of, I would say, yes, at the very least because the matter affects the modes of cooperativity that are possible. Now notice the difference in what I am saying from what Searle said when he said that 'only brains can think'. I am saying there may be something about the biophysics of brains which makes them the embodiment of conscious thinking in a sense in which things with imposed structure, even with all these embellishments, may not be. It's an open question – an empirical question in principle.

Finally let me insist that I am not going back on the suggestion that we have been following through in this book that what identifies you or me is the information-flow system in which we are each embodied with our respective states of conditional readiness. No, what I am suggesting is that the physical basis of our state of conditional readiness may extend downwards to sub-microscopic levels as yet beyond our ken and certainly beyond our understanding. It is for this reason that I would regard the possibility of artificial agents that can be conscious as a genuinely open question.

Producing conscious agents: the Creator's prerogative?

If anyone imagines that by entertaining this I am open to the objection that the production artificially of a conscious human-like agent would usurp the prerogative of the Creator I would suggest that this objection would be a confusion between the theological notion of creation, which is the giving of being to what *is*, and procreation, which is what we all have a divine licence to do (if we believe in the theistic position at all). Procreation is the reassembly of components of the physical world in a process that we may not understand but which results in the coming into being of an organization which embodies a new centre of conscious awareness: there is somebody there at the end of it. If procreation can, in this science fiction context, be successfully accomplished by means other than the normal pleasurable process, then this may be surprising to most of us, including me, but it seems to me it is totally devoid of the theological conclusion that we have usurped the prerogative of the Creator.

Notes

1 In the post-lecture discussion the actual words were: '... whether that organism over there – [to the chairman] will you do, sir? – is conscious. ... There would be one individual, I put it to you, who would know we are wrong on a matter of fact, and that would be our chairman.'

⑨

My Fault or My Brain's?

The 'doctrine of necessity'

I would like to introduce our topic, and perhaps clarify it, with a well-known quotation from the lawyer Clarence Darrow, who once addressed the prisoners in the Cook County jail in the following words:

> There is no such thing as a crime as the word is generally understood. I do not believe there is any sort of distinction between the real moral conditions of the people in and out of jail. One is just as good as the other. The people here can no more help being here than the people outside can avoid being outside. I do not believe that people are in jail because they deserve to be. They are in jail simply because they cannot avoid it on account of circumstances which are *entirely beyond their control* and for which they are in no way responsible. . . . There are people who think that everything in this world is an accident. But really there is no such thing as an accident. . . . There are a great many people here who have done some of these things (murder, theft, etc.) who really do not know themselves why they did them. It looked to you at the time as if you had a chance to do them or not, as you saw fit; but still, *after all you had no choice.* . . . If you look at the question deeply enough and carefully enough you will see that there were circumstances that *drove you* to do exactly the thing which you did. *You could not help it* any more than we outside can help taking the positions that we take. (My italics.)

That is a fairly robust statement of a point of view which is, of course, not novel with Clarence Darrow. It goes back many centuries. Indeed it was the danger that this point of view would follow from Democritus's theory of atomism in the time of the ancient Greeks, that led Epicurus to make some cosmetic emendations suggesting that the atoms batting about in the void might sometimes make tiny swerves which would be enough to allow room for free will.

It is on this kind of view that the great Thomas Reid, who succeeded Adam Smith to the chair of philosophy in the University of Glasgow, had some characteristically common sense things to say:

> All conviction of wrong conduct, all remorse and self-condemnation, imply a conviction of our power to have done better. Take away this conviction, and there may be a sense of misery, or a dread of evil to come, but there can be no sense of guilt, or resolution to do better.
>
> Many who hold the doctrine of necessity, disown these consequences of it, and think to evade them ... but ... some late patrons of it have had the boldness to avow them. 'They cannot accuse themselves of having done anything wrong in the ultimate sense of the words. In a strict sense, they have nothing to do with repentance, confession, and pardon, these being adapted to a fallacious view of things.'
>
> Those who can adopt these sentiments, may indeed celebrate, with high encomiums, *the great and glorious doctrine of necessity*. It restores them, in their own conceit, to the state of innocence. It delivers them from all the pangs of guilt and remorse, and from all fear about their future conduct, though not about their fate. They may be as secure that they shall do nothing wrong, as those who have finished their course. A doctrine so flattering to the mind of a sinner, is very apt to give strength to weak arguments.

Facts about ourselves

Now we want, of course, to face as squarely as possible all the *facts* about ourselves that we have available. From the start of this book I have been emphasizing the strong demand on our thinking of two different categories of fact. First are the facts of my conscious experience, which include the fact that I can and do, sometimes, find myself able to determine, by thinking, valuing and selecting, my course of action. (There are also all the other facts of my conscious experience that I would be lying to deny.) Secondly, there are the facts that we have been following through in some detail: the facts of physiology and brain science which seem to indicate that our brain must be thought of as a physical system subject to laws similar to those which we find reliable in the rest of the physical world.

We have been using a summary form of analysis of the complexity of

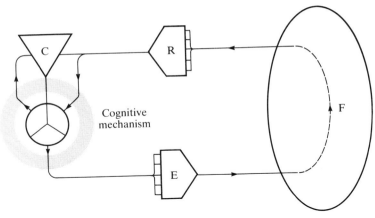

Figure 9.1   The representation of what an agent knows: simplified form of information-flow map of an agent which sets its own goals for activity in its world of action. The agent's representation of its world is contained within its cognitive mechanism.

the real brain, and to focus our thinking we can make use of it again in this chapter. We have built up a flow system such as figure 7.1, which we are supposing to be embodied in our brains in something of the way in which, say, the trade system of the world is embodied in the economic community of the world. It showed in a little detail the sequence of indication, evaluation and selection of action in view of a goal – the goal itself being selected by a meta-organizing system in view of evaluation of the current success of the ongoing interaction with the world. In chapter 7 we simplified the diagram down to figure 7.2: we collapsed the organizing and meta-organizing systems into a central structure representing, among other things, the facts believed, the skills acquired and the norms – indeed the hierarchy of norms, the priority scheme – which govern the setting of goals by the individual in his field of action.

For our present purpose I am going to use an even simpler labelling scheme where we can say that the whole of the region concerned with *what we know and believe* deserves a single name of the *cognitive mechanism* (figure 9.1). This doesn't mean that every aspect of it is equally related to conscious cognition, but it does mean, among other things, that no change can take place in what the agent believes to be the case without a change taking place somewhere within this cognitive mechanism. When I say this, you will remember that I insisted earlier that this was not dogma. It is a working assumption. But our purpose now is to ask what its consequences would be. I imagine that it is very much the kind of working assumption that a man like Clarence Darrow might have had in mind in making that sweeping statement of his with which we began. Insofar as brain science has followed through this kind of sequence, it finds no reason to doubt a causal linkage along each of the lines of this diagram. Its model is, for practical purposes, a deterministic model – except that there is room, as I mentioned in the previous chapter, for a probabilistic or stochastic element when it comes to some of the fine details of the cognitive mechanism.

Let us assume determinacy of toughest sort

For the present I am going to ask us to postpone discussion of the possibility that some of the cognitive mechanism might function probabilistically or indeterministically. We are going to set ourselves the toughest case: we are going to be asking, what *if* – and it is a strongly underlined if – the whole of this system as summarized here were a determinate system in the physical sense? That is to say, if every physical event had its adequate determinants in other and earlier physical events, would it follow (as the Darrows of the world appear to think) that we have no choice, everything is inevitable, and we couldn't have done otherwise?

What do we mean by 'inevitable'?

Let us begin clarifying what we are going to mean by these hypothetical statements by considering some standard examples where we *would* say we 'don't have any option'. Take, for example, the times of sunset printed in our diaries. That sunset at Glasgow will be at a certain time tomorrow is indeed something that we would all say is inevitable for us; there is nothing we can do about it. It is not something that we can be blamed for. There exists a specification of the time of sunset such that anyone and everyone would be correct to believe it and incorrect to reject it. This notion of statements which have an *uncondi-*

tional claim to assent is basic enough to be worth our writing out (as the bottom line of table 9.2). What we are trying to do is to compare other statements about ourselves as to the strength of *their* claims to assent. Notice that what we are discussing is a logical concept and not a psychological one. We are not asking: how plausible does this sound, or would we be able to persuade somebody to assent to it? What we are asking is: is the strength of the statement 'the sun will set at a certain time tomorrow' such that it has a claim to your assent and mine which is *unconditional*? Another way of putting it is to say: is the event described *inevitable for us*? And of course to this question of sunset we would normally say: yes, given the assumptions of deterministic astronomy.

A rigid prediction of an agent's future

Now what would follow if this flow system we have been considering were a deterministic system? In particular, what would follow with respect to the cognitive mechanism? (Your cognitive mechanism, you remember, is where you store what you know.) Well, it would follow that there would be a specification, 'CM', of the state of the cognitive mechanism (and in principle this is something which has a claim to the assent of, let us say, a super-scientist who is observing the mechanism with appropriate equipment, but who does not convey any information back to the agent, A). This would be a specification with implications not merely for the present moment, but also for the immediate future. If it is a deterministic system, then from the current state there follows a description, for at least the immediate future, given that the environment interacting with the system is itself deterministic. So we are being very classical for the moment, from a physical angle. We are imagining that for practical purposes the system is as deterministic as the solar system and could in principle give rise to specifications of that sort for the cognitive mechanism. There is going to be no drawing back on this: if the system is deterministic then the super-observer who tells the O-story (the outside story about our brains) will obtain this specification CM(t) and will have to recognize that it has an unconditional claim to his assent – just like statements about the times of sunset for the astronomer.

Who else would be correct to believe CM(t)?

Now we ask: what does this imply for the agent, A, whose brain we are talking about? Perhaps to make this quite clear we will redraw our old diagram, table 1.1, with slight modification to the headings of our two columns (table 9.1). A is the name of the agent who tells the I-story about his conscious mental life. We are now going to talk about the second column in more general terms than 'brain': it is the O-story, the story that an outside observer with full scientific information would be committed to. This will, as before, be something to do with brain activity, neural states x, y, z and so on. In particular, the correlate of the statement 'I believe such and such' will be a particular fact about some part of the cognitive mechanism, as indicated in the right-hand column. By this we mean that no change could take place in what you, the agent, believe without a change in your state of conditional readiness (as we called it) which is embodied in the cognitive mechanism. So the cognitive mechanism contains the correlate of any fact you believe. Not that it is a one to one correspondence. We pointed out that there might be a number of alternative physical configurations which were equivalent as regards conditional readiness, and therefore there might be several physical conditions each of which would represent the fact that you believe that 13 is a prime number, or that today is Thursday, or whatever. But in general there is that strong correlation, in that no change can take place in what

Table 9.1 The correlated inside and outside accounts of a conscious agent's mental activity

A the agent tells the I-story	O the observer tells the brain-story
I see . . .	Neural activity x
I hear . . .	Neural activity y
I like . . .	Neural s_1
I believe . . .	Neural state s_2
etc.	etc.

The region within the box contains the neural correlates of all that the agent knows and believes. This region is the cognitive mechanism, CM.

you believe without a change taking place in your cognitive mechanism.

The O-story about the present and immediately future state of the cognitive mechanism of A is being told by (or could in principle be told by) the super-observer, O, who has access to all the information necessary to make his predictions. But what about A? What can A say about the story, CM(t), which has an unconditional claim to the assent of O? Shouldn't he be correct to believe it too – or at least shouldn't he wish he knew it in order to believe it? And the answer which we have already encountered (in chapter 5) is: no, on the contrary, there is the strongest logical reason for A's not believing CM(t) because CM(t) is accurate in relation to the *present* state of his cognitive mechanism. If A were to believe CM(t), or if any change were to take place in A's cognitive mechanism, then CM(t) would no longer be accurate. There can be no complete specification of CM(t) which is equally accurate whether or not A believes it. (Note that we are talking here only about A's cognitive mechanism and not about *everything* that happens to A in the future. Not only for the times of sunset, but also for lots of other things that can happen to human beings there can exist universally valid predictions with an unconditional claim on all.)

'Disclaim' to assent

The specification which is valid for O is untruthful for A, in that if A believed it the changes in A's cognitive mechanism would make it out of date and false. This brought out what we called the principle of logical relativity. This is that what O is correct to believe about A's cognitive mechanism is precisely what A would be incorrect to believe if only he knew it.

Oddly enough, then, the specification of A's cognitive mechanism CM(t), which has an unconditional claim to the assent of O, the observer, has no unconditional claim to the assent of A, the agent. Indeed it has a 'disclaim' to A's assent. We are not talking about whether A could be persuaded to believe it or anything like that. We are simply saying that as a matter of logical fact it does not have a logical claim to A's assent. It guarantees that A would be mistaken to believe it.

Well that's odd; but it has to be faced and we have to ask what can be salvaged from it. Certainly we are not denying that A, in retrospect, if shown a cine film tomorrow of O's evidence, can agree that O was correct. He can agree that CM(t) was an accurate prediction from O's standpoint. So A *in retrospect* does not deny that O was right in believing CM(t). But equally O in retrospect does not deny and cannot deny that A would have been in error to believe CM(t). The relativistic situation is inescapable; but it doesn't prevent A, the agent, from believing that (of course unknown to him) O has a belief which in due course will turn out to have been correct.

The odd thing – but the thing that we must cling on to and do justice to – is that A can say this without at all implying that he was ignorant of 'the truth'. Because, of course, what he is ignorant of is something that would be *un*truthful for him. He would be in error to believe it. So we can say that CM(t) is unbeliefworthy for A even if it has an unconditional claim to O's assent. Both of these things are *true* of CM(t).

Perhaps I can take you back again to one of the demonstrations of chapter 1 and say a little more about it. What we were trying to do then was to make a TV camera produce a picture of its own screen. If you do this, what you see on the screen is an artefact produced by the feedback from screen to camera, and if you zoom the camera in you reach a point where the whole thing goes into shimmering confusion reflecting the fact that there cannot – logically cannot – be a picture which is equally accurate whether or not the camera is trying to depict it. There is no picture of a picture which can be stable if the picture is trying to depict itself. Instead the 'solution to the equation', so to speak, is logically indeterminate and the best a physical system can do is to oscillate between various possible solutions.

On the other hand, if we now go a step further and go right in to as big a magnification as possible, an interesting thing happens. We can now look at the individual pixels on the screen, the individual specks of light and dark, and you see that it is possible – give or take a bit of flicker – for the system to work again. Because now we are using the whole depicting mechanism to represent only a tiny part of itself. So there is nothing in principle to prevent the selection of parts of a depictive system to be represented more or less accurately in different parts, other parts, of the depictive mechanism. Provided you can segregate the two systems and not try to make a representation of the state of affairs which is itself to be the representation, then you are not in a logical bind.

By the same token, there are many things which it is perfectly possible in principle for the agent A to know and believe, even about the immediate future of his cognitive mechanism. So we are not saying that everything about his brain must be equally indeterminate for him. But what we can say is that certainly there must be some aspects of the state of his cognitive mechanism which are not merely unknowable by him, but indeterminate for him. You see the distinction? Talking about unknowability is talking about how easily he could get access. We are not talking about that. What we are saying is that even if he could get access it has no determinative function for him. Its selective function is not singular. It is ill-defined. It is indeterminate. It is untrustworthy by him, unbeliefworthy by him. Yet this is compatible with saying that the immediate future of his cognitive mechanism is predictable in principle by a detached observer. Now this is very odd, I can't deny it.

Logical indeterminacy

Human beings are a quite extraordinary category of object in the world. For all the other objects in the world we have reason to believe, give or take Heisenberg's uncertainty principle, that there *does* exist, whether we know it or not, one and only one picture of the immediate future such that anyone and everyone would be correct to believe it and mistaken to disbelieve it. But of the little piece of matter inside your head, wherever it is in that structure, which embodies your state of conditional readiness, *there does not exist* any such specification unknown to us with a unique and unequivocal claim to the assent of everyone if only they knew it. This needs a word, and I have suggested that we call the immediate future of A's cognitive mechanism *logically indeterminate*. So we have got logical indeterminacy here – using the word logical (it is not perhaps the best term) to differentiate it from physical indeterminacy because *this* indeterminacy, the absence of a definitive specification with a universal claim to the assent of all, is compatible with physical determinism. So it could be physically determinate and still what I have called logically indeterminate.

Allowing for the effects of telling the agent the prediction

Now you may reasonably object that I have so far been talking about a case where O, the observer, simply sticks to his calculations based on the current state. And you might say, couldn't he doctor his prediction in such a way as to allow for the effects of A's believing it? Now if we do start asking that, we are talking about something quite different. We are talking about an *experimental* situation where somebody actually feeds A with predictions. But never mind, let's follow through the implications. What we are saying is, let O make a calculation which corrects his prediction CM(t) into something else, which we will call $CM_1(t)$. This is a revised prediction which allows for the effects that A's believing it would have on A's cognitive mechanism. You get the idea: O adjusts, so as to compensate for the inaccuracies that would otherwise be introduced by A's believing it. O has now come up (if it is possible) with a specification that *can* claim A's assent. Assuming that the calculation can be done (and that is not obvious, but assuming for the sake of argument that it can), $CM_1(t)$ is a prediction designed to be accurate *if and only if* A believes it. All right, so A would not be in error to believe $CM_1(t)$. But let us ask the other question which every logician would insist on: would A be in error to *dis*believe it?

We have allowed O to produce his adapted prediction in a form which he can claim would be correct if and only if A believed it. But it *is* 'if-and-only-if' and it follows from that that an A who disbelieved $CM_1(t)$ would not be in error. Because $CM_1(t)$ will not be accurate for *anybody* unless A believes it! So that A, from a logical standpoint, is as entitled to disbelieve $CM_1(t)$ as to believe it. All that O has succeeded in doing by his clever trickery is to come up with a formula which A would be equally correct to accept or reject. Indeed the accuracy of $CM_1(t)$ depends precisely on whether A believes it or not. So in the strongest possible sense A's cognitive attitude to $CM_1(t)$ determines the accuracy of $CM_1(t)$ – or if you like determines the immediate future of his cognitive mechanism.

So all that we have done by following through this imaginary loophole is to demonstrate yet again that there does not exist one and only one specification of the immediate future of your cognitive mechanism with an unconditional claim to your assent. There is nothing unconditional about the claim to assent of $CM_1(t)$; it is some-

thing that indeed you would be correct to believe, but it is also something that you would be correct to disbelieve. As it happens, there is
an American idiom that makes this point quite nicely. You offer an
American a tray with tea and coffee and in certain parts of the States
the idiom would be 'I believe I'll have some tea'. By saying 'I believe I
will have some tea', he makes it the case that he will have tea. Or he
may say 'I believe I have had enough tea, I'll have coffee', and by
believing that he will not have tea he makes it the case that he will not
have tea.

Not even the most physically deterministic model of the cognitive
process and its workings and connections can come up with a prediction of the immediate future of your cognitive mechanism with an
unconditional claim to your assent. In that sense then there is a stark
contrast between even this adapted case and the case of predictions of
eclipses and things of that sort in the physical world. Brains are
different from everything else in the physical world in that the strongest
possible claim you can generate for a prediction of their immediate
future is one that the agent in question would be equally correct to
accept or reject. He is no more in a bind of inevitability *vis-à-vis*
$CM_1(t)$ than you would be if two urchins were to come in from the
street and offer you two bits of paper on one of which is written 'you
will take tea' and on the other 'you will not take tea'. One of them is
going to be correct – that's analytic, that's trivial – but there is
nothing binding about either of them as far as you are concerned. And
the same is true of $CM_1(t)$.

An agent's future is open to him

Let us sum up for the moment. As A, the agent, contemplates his
future he is correct to believe that no single determinate specification
exists, unknown to him, with an unconditional claim to *his* assent if
only he knew it. ('Correct' here means warranted by all the facts
known, or rather assumed, by us: determinism and all the rest.) The
future specification of A's cognitive mechanism is open and
undetermined for him in a way that the future of the solar system or
any other part of the physically determinate world is not. It is a future
that *waits to be determined* by what he thinks or decides. So we have got
yet another angle on the efficacy, the 'causal efficacy' as some would
call it, certainly the determinative efficacy of mental activity.

How do random events affect our freedom?

Now note here the contrast with a mere absence of physical determinacy. I promised to lift the embargo on the assumption of determinism: let us do it now. What if indeed we bring Heisenberg uncertainty into the physical picture? Then I think we are in an area where we have to recognize that many chains of entailment that an engineer might draw down through the cognitive mechanism might fail to carry through because of 'random fluctuation'. I say 'many': there is no knowing how many, but let us suppose that at least occasionally there would be some. What good would this do in facing the issue raised by Darrow and addressed in very different terms by Reid?

Let's begin with the solar system. Suppose the solar system proved, as indeed it may, to have ingredients of its determinants that are indeterminate from the standpoint of physics. Would this make its future any less inevitable for you? No, it would not give you any advantage in facing the time of sunrise tomorrow to know that it might fluctuate randomly. Physical indeterminism as such is worthless as an ameliorator of the apparent problem of facing a future that looks inevitable. To make it an indeterminate future means that you have yet another factor outside your control. So mere randomness or indeterminacy introduced into the works of the brain would, I suggest, be no answer at all to the problem that Thomas Reid, for example, has highlighted so clearly. What matters first and foremost is that the immediate future of the cognitive mechanism, which we are assuming to be among the main determinants of action, *is* determined, in part at least, by A's thinking and the like. And *then* of course, given that, we must check that it has no determinate specification already with an unconditional claim to A's assent, in other words that it is still open to A to determine.

Embodiment and determination

We looked earlier at this way of talking in the case of a computer. To say that the computer is solving Laplace's equation, or whatever, is (among other things) to claim that its behaviour is *determined by* Laplace's equation; but nobody in his senses imagines that this means that there is a ghostly entity, the equation, hovering and influencing random or other processes in the computer in addition to the forces that physics recognizes within the transistors and other components. Why? Because the equation is not an additional entity interacting with the physical system. It is a mathematical entity, if you like, *embodied in* the system. The notion of embodiment is crucial.

What makes our thinking the determinant of our cognitive mechanism's immediate future, I suggest, is that our thinking is embodied in the processes that we have been looking at in the previous few chapters, the processes which are diagrammed in abstract in the flow map of figure 9.1. The argument I have spelt out in this chapter merely reinforces this: the notion that physical determinism (if admitted) would block off the possibility that cognitive activity could determine the future of CM is itself fallacious.

Freedom of action

Of course you recognize now that this applies not merely to the immediate future of the cognitive mechanism but also to the immediate future of the whole system, insofar as its form is shaped by the state of the cognitive mechanism. Actions are characteristically activities selected in view of ends. To the extent that actions are selected by way of cognitive machinery of this sort, they share in the logical indeterminacy of the cognitive mechanism itself. It is as true of actions (those actions suitably coupled, as to cause, with the cognitive mechanism) as it is of the cognitive mechanism's own future, that they *have no unique determinate specification* in advance of your making up your mind and taking them.

That is, they have no determinate unique specification with an unconditional claim to *your* assent, even though they may, in our imaginary science fiction world, have a claim to the assent of the observer O which *is* unconditional. He, if he is (as it were) behind a one-way screen and totally isolated from any possibility of interfering with you, may, as a spectator, witness the determinative processes in your cognitive net and come to the conclusion that you are about to decline the cup of tea. There is nothing whatever in that, so far, which implies that, willy-nilly, it is inevitable for *you* that you are about to refuse the cup of tea. Quite the contrary: the same data which O would appeal to, to justify his expectation that you will indeed refuse the cup of tea, will also allow O to insist that for you the possibility is still open, to have it and not have it, and that his belief would immediately be ruined as to its cognitive claim if you were to attempt to believe it, because you would not then be in the state which his calculation pre-supposed.

What we are saying is that the openness of the domain of action, which we in common sense would bear witness to, is undergirded and not in the least undermined by considerations of the details of the mechanistic embodiment of the thinking that determines the actions.

Could I have done otherwise?

In particular, the question 'could I have done otherwise?' must now be clearly separated (in a way that regrettably many classical articles on the subject do not) from the question: 'could my *brain* have gone through different motions as viewed by O?' These are two radically separate questions. That is perhaps the main point that I want to make. You will find reams of literature in the philosophical journals on the question 'could I have done otherwise?', and they nearly always confuse two questions. The needle jumps the groove from the question 'could *I* have done otherwise?' (which is an I-story question using the categories of the I-story) to the O-story question 'could my *brain* (as viewed of course from the standpoint of O) have been expected to have gone through other motions?'

What I have tried to show, and what I believe is inescapable, is that you can answer 'yes' to the one and 'no' to the other. And that indeed there is a certain complementarity between the yes answer (where the contents of column 1 of table 9.1 are concerned) and the no answer (respecting some parts of column 2). Certainly the data of the brain-story reinforce the correctness of the I-story answer.

So I am suggesting that if we are going to make sense of the question of what is classically known as 'free will' by asking, for example, whether I could have done otherwise if my brain were a physically determinate system, we must not at any cost allow ourselves to confuse that with the question: could my *brain* have done otherwise. The reason is that it is not brains but persons who choose, persons who have I-stories to tell. There is no sense that I can see in attributing free will to brains: brains aren't the kind of things, poor objects, to have free will. But persons certainly are, at least they are claimants. We have then two questions, not one:

1   Was there more than one specification of my future action each of which could have had an open claim to my assent, that is, each of which I would have been equally correct to accept? That is the one question: which is a spelling out of 'could *I* have done otherwise?'

2   Was there more than one specification of my future *brain state* each of which could have an equally valid claim to O's assent? To that question the answer of a deterministic neurophysiology would be no. Even if we go to indeterminate physiology (which I think is realistic for reasons that I sketched in the previous chapter and will be talking about again later) the additional uncertainty introduced by the stochastic, probabilistic element in the functioning of the brain would not, as I see it, increase significantly my claim to have had a share in determining my action. It might increase the frustration of the observer, O, in trying to predict it. But I have been arguing, perhaps now *ad nauseam*, that that is irrelevant. Because we can grant it 100 per cent. It is irrelevant to the question of the openness to you, as agent, of the range of actions which you contemplate in trying to take a decision.

[*Where does this take us as regards Clarence Darrow?*] What Darrow could argue is that from the standpoint of a fully informed observer, the causal chain-mesh leading up to the crime might have been fully predictable. What Darrow concludes from this (jumping over into the I-story) is that the *agent* had no option, that there was nothing open to him other than what he did, that he could not help it, that it was outside his range of control. Every one of these I am trying to show in detail is false, simply false, a blunder.

What the evidence of O shows is merely and strictly – and of course non-trivially – that the criminal action was predictable by O. It does not show that it was inevitable for A, the agent – unless (see below) it can be shown that the causality was of a kind which by-passed the cognitive mechanism in such a way as to make the prediction that led to the action have an unconditional claim to that agent's assent. That's my argument: and it is of course a point totally missed by Darrow.

Diminished responsibility

Now I have said all this on the assumption that the system is functioning normally. I ought, of course, to point out that brains can go wrong. As a result of drugs, anatomical malfunction, failure of blood supply and many other causes, there are unfortunate people in the world whose cognitive processes do not determine their actions with the kind of reliability that ours normally do. It is interesting to notice that it is the *failure* of determination which, in terms of this argument at least, makes it rational for us to diminish the degree of responsibility which we attribute to them. In other words, determinism, insofar as it is identifiable, is a help to the attribution of responsibility.

The person who needs to be denied responsibility – a measure which, when you think about it, is a terrible insult to any cognitive agent – is the person for whose total system some of the normal determining links have broken down. If, for instance, the coupling between the indicative and the normative process has broken down (between the segments marked 'maps' and 'norms' in figure 7.2) then you will have somebody who could in principle be told the outcome of a choice situation you are about to put him through, and the telling would, because of the breakdown of the coupling, have no causal influence on the normative process. For such an individual the outcome would be inevitable. A simple example would be the extreme one of sticking an electrode into someone else's brain and electrifying the region of the brain that would normally receive its electrical input from his cognitive mechanism. You say 'your arm is about to rise', and you press the button and his arm does rise. The knowledge you have given, in the specification of the immediate future, is true knowledge for the agent because the poor agent has had a breakdown between his cognitive and executive system.

So you see that the argument I have been sketching does not in the least imply that *every* act by a human being must be equally attributed to what traditionally would be called his 'free choice'. There could certainly be situations, especially in cases of drugs, epilepsy, failure of blood supply, Parkinson's disease and who knows what else, where the agent would be not merely entitled to plead that 'he couldn't help it', he would be backed up by the O-story account that would be given of the breakdown in his cognitive mechanism. But – and this is the point – it would not be on the ground that the story is deterministic, because the other stories, which I have insisted *do not* invalidate the claim to responsibility, are also deterministic. Fastening on the degree of determinism is fastening on the wrong thing. That is what I want to insist particularly. It is not a question of whether the mechanism is deterministic. It is a question of what kind of determinative chain is involved: does it by-pass the cognitive mechanism? If it does, then you must deny the individual some share of responsibility *pro rata*. If it doesn't then insofar as these considerations follow, he is *entitled* – it is not a matter of something you force on him – he cannot escape, as a matter of entitlement, the praise or blame for doing the action as the agent.

The only rational grounds on which Darrow could deny the criminal the dignity of being blamed for the crime would be evidence, from the mechanical analysis, that the causal chain-mesh by-passed the agent's cognitive mechanism so that – whatever the agent thought about it, however he wished, however he valued – it was going to come that way any way. But that is not the case Darrow is talking about.

Another way of putting it is that, if you spell out the counter-factuals which are implicit in the Darrow scenario, they are not supported by the evidence in the case of a normal brain. *If* the 'criminal' had an epileptic seizure of a certain sort which threw him into a violent rage and so forth . . . then that, maybe, is the category that we are talking about where the normal route through the cognitive mechanism was by-passed. But that is not, of course, what Darrow is on about: he is on about the whole population of Cook County jail. And he is, I would say, offering an affront to the dignity of most of them, and in a manner which is quite unwarranted by even the most deterministic model of the causality of brain processes.

Indeterminacy of a community to itself

Another point, which I touched on in an earlier context, is that in a community of individuals in dialogue this indeterminacy is mutual. If there is more than one agent in dialogue with one other then each knows the other as, to some extent, an indeterminate agent. Not in the sense that he doesn't happen to know what the future actions will be, but that *there does not exist* one and only one unique and determinate specification of the other's actions which, if only he knew it, he would be correct unconditionally to accept. All members of the group are not merely entitled, but logically bound to recognize the others with whom they are in dialogue, as determining agents facing a future which is indeterminate for all of them until they individually and/or collectively make up their minds.

And this is, of course, what human beings do in the world in which we attribute responsibility to one another. Attribution of responsibility is characteristically communal. It has to do with the rationality of answering the question: why did you do that? Any member of a community is entitled to ask it. And the point of my argument is that there is nothing whatever irrational or contrary to mechanistic brain science in this practice. Indeed what I am saying is that the rationality of the practice of blaming, contrary to Darrow, does not at all depend upon denying physical determinism, or 'necessity' to use Reid's phrase.

'Beyond his control' . . .

Whether a particular event X was outside A's control is, as we saw even when we thought about servo-systems, a technical factual question. Some things are outside our control and some are not and you can look at the flow map to find out which are and which are not and it is nothing whatever to do with whether our mechanism, in and through which we are embodied as determinative agents, is a physically determinate structure.

. . . And 'of necessity'?

I have to say that this relativistic point, this distinction, is not a point that you will find in Reid or indeed in many (or any) of the discussions of this dilemma. Reid refers to the doctrine of necessity as 'a great and glorious doctrine' ironically (i.e. with his tongue in his cheek), but as an unambiguous concept. One way of putting the argument I have set before you is that this is not an unambiguous concept.

The doctrine of necessity *is* ambiguous and it has two forms. One is the doctrine that in the physical world, including the world of the brain, every event has an adequate and determining physical cause. Now that may or may not be true: Heisenberg's principle sets doubts against it. That is one kind of doctrine; it is a doctrine about the way the physical structure works. The other doctrine of necessity, in the way that Reid and Darrow have been talking about it classically, is equivalent to the doctrine of inevitability. It is the doctrine that if you assume that the system is physically determinate then the immediate future is 'inevitable'. But that does not follow, as I have shown. On the contrary, your brain could be as mechanical as the solar system, as physically determinate as the solar system, and yet your immediate future is not inevitable for you or those in dialogue with you, in the sense in which the future of the solar system is.

The 'cerebroscope'

It may be felt that I devised this argument in order to arrive at a position which I wished, on other grounds, to uphold. In fact, historically, I came at it from quite a different direction. In the late 1940s a small group of scientists with a common interest in brain mechanics began to meet for informal discussions at the National Hospital in London. It called itself the Ratio Club, and A. M. Turing, Horace Barlow and some 20 others were members. Some of us were interested in electrical recording from the brain, and at one of our sessions (I think in 1952) I presented a curious paradox that I had stumbled across by asking what would happen if I were able to use what I called a 'cerebroscope' to study the workings of my own brain. It became clear that there would be one region of the brain which would not merely be unobservable by me, but which could not have a specification with an unconditional claim to my assent. All that I have been saying in this chapter follows from that. I think it is unassailable – it has not been assailed in the past 30 years. And if it is unassailable, then we've got to face it. It has the very interesting consequence that it enables one to see the fallacy in the Clarence Darrow type of argument, and also (below) in some of the classical debates over divine sovereignty as well.

God's knowledge of our futures

Finally we come back to a question that has surfaced more than once and is perhaps germane to the concerns of the Gifford lectureship as much as any. It is the objection that we are leaving God out of account. Now it is not my place or my brief to advocate belief in God. But it is a very fair question that if you did believe in God, would you not then have to say that God at least knows my future? Surely everything God knows is the truth and therefore we are in theological trouble. I would like briefly to say why I think that is not the case.

I accept the tough-minded concept of God as the Author of all that is. (I think you can have all kinds of weak concepts of God to make things easy in philosophical discussions of this sort. But for our purpose and, as a matter of fact, personally I accept the more tough-minded concept of God as the Author of all that is.) So let us take that as the doctrine whose consequences we are spelling out, just as we took physical determinism in its extreme form.

Aquinas has put it that 'God's knowledge is the cause of the future'. I am not entirely happy with the word 'cause' but certainly one could follow him in comparing the dependence of our world on God in the theistic sense with the dependence of a created world on the author-ship of a human being. If a human being is the author of a creation then there is a direct relation between at least the creative say-so, the *fiat*, of the author and every feature in that world. And the moment you say that, you realize that divine sovereignty, which follows from it (as Aquinas insists, just as strongly as Calvin ever did) has *nothing to do* with physical determinism. That is important. If the divine Being is being conceived of as the Author of all that is, as a novelist is the author of all that is in a novel, the doctrine of divine sovereignty implies that there are no events – but no events – in the created order other than according to the author's say-so. If it is the author's whim that some of those events are random, in the sense that the inhabitants of the world find no causal precursors for them and could find none because there are none, that does not make them any less directly dependent upon the sovereignty of the author. There is nothing to stop you or me from writing a novel in which events in a Geiger counter or something like that have no causal precursors. It is up to the author.

So point number one is that we must not confuse doctrines of divine sovereignty with physical theories of determinism in physics. Here, although there is not space to go into it, I am afraid I am running counter to quite a lot of recent popular theological literature, from the Archbishop of York (John Habgood) and others, which talks about God as not having sovereignty over the random components of his world but 'building-in randomness as a tool' and so on. It is all right to talk like that, but I am describing it as a softer concept of God than the one which Aquinas, for example, recognizes to be the theistic one of the Bible. And as I shall be arguing in a moment, I don't see any rational pressure to move in that direction.

Describing to us our immediately future state: can God do it?

Since these points we have been considering are logical points they must apply as strongly to those propositions or specifications that we imagine God as entertaining as to those of anyone else. In other words, if God is the Author of the whole on-going show, in which your cognitive mechanism is about to go into a particular state CM(t), then of course in the sense in which an author knows the content of his novel, God knows the state CM(t). But the author (and you can think of this in terms of a human author if you like) would be the first to insist that what he knows about the immediate future of his characters is not something these characters could be correct to believe. Obvious, isn't it, because a character who believed it would not be the character of whom the story was written. Perhaps John in your novel asks Mary to marry him and Mary has a sleepless night and then decides to say yes. The fact that Mary decides to say yes is something you as author know timelessly relative to the whole space–time you have created, but it is certainly not a proposition with an unconditional claim to Mary's assent during her sleepless night. A Mary who believed it would not be the Mary who had a sleepless night wondering whether to make it the case or not. This is hardly an original point but you see what I am saying. You don't do any credit to the omnipotent God by predicating of Him the power to make a logical self-contradiction.

Even God, as I see it, even the author God with the total divine sovereignty of classical theism, could not specify the immediate future of your cognitive mechanism in such a form that you would be correct to believe it and in error to disbelieve it. This is important and we shall be coming back to it. (Note that I am not saying that it would be impossible for God-in-dialogue with man to make any predictions. That would be nonsense, of course. It is only predictions of the cognitive mechanism that are ruled out.)

If, then, we take seriously the concept of dialogue with God, even God in dialogue with us meets us and knows us as determinators. He knows us as determinators of an immediate future which is indeterminate, notice, both for us *and* for Him in dialogue with us. For one who comes into dialogue with a cognitive agent – and dialogue means of course a reciprocal relation involving the cognitive mechanism of that agent – is in a situation in which there does not exist one and only one specification of the total situation with an unconditional claim to the assent of either of them.

The Creator-Participant: projections of God's being

As soon as you say *that*, you recognize that by taking seriously the concept of dialogue with God, you have made untenable any single Person model of the Deity. This I think is non-trivial. Speak of the Deity as the Author of space–time – and you can use personal categories, of course, as the Bible does and as classical theistic theology does – and you are speaking of the Person of the Creator. But speak of God as One who can enter into dialogue with His created agents, and you are speaking of One for whom the knowledge He will have of those with whom He enters into dialogue is not the knowledge of the Creator outside the space–time He has created. Or to put it the other way round, the One in dialogue with agents in space–time logically cannot have the knowledge which the Author outside space–time (for whom space–time is one fact) can have.

So, interestingly enough, by following through the logical implications of the concept of dialogue, we reach the conclusion that if we are to have a theology in which there is any room for dialogue with God, we cannot have a model of God simplified to a single Person. We need at least two personal projections of the being of God if we are to do justice to the two aspects of what we are attributing to the Deity.

This, I think, is a point which unties some of the knots that have classically been drawn tight around the concepts of divine sovereignty and human responsibility. One of the classical discussions of our freedom *vis-à-vis* God is that in which Lorenzo Valla imagines an antagonist who says: 'What would you think, if God having truly predicted my action, were to predict it to me?' Lorenzo's only answer is: 'Believe me, you who thus lie in wait to deceive God, if you should hear or certainly know what He said you would do, either out of love, or out of fear you would hasten to do what you knew was predicted by Him.' I see this as an evasion, I'm afraid, and an unnecessary one. Unnecessary, because the answer which emerges from the above analysis appears to be that the knowledge which is properly predicable of the Creator in eternity (technically called 'fore-knowledge', the 'fore' being gratuitous) would not *be* knowledge for the Deity in dialogue with you. Therefore the question doesn't arise. The One who, in dialogue with you, would challenge you, in the way that Lorenzo imagines God challenging the other, would not be the same Person as the One of whom classical theism predicates fore-knowledge.

Summary

I have argued that responsibility for our choices, whether to our fellows or to God, does not depend upon denying physical determinism in the human brain. If you take physical determinism in even its strictest and strongest form, it turns out logically *not* to imply what many people have supposed it did: namely the existence of one, and only one, specification of your future state, with an unconditional claim to be beliefworthy by you, if only you knew it, or sufficient to prove that you were under an illusion if you do not believe it. On the contrary, we found a rather interesting logical situation which is summarized in table 9.2.

We have been talking about the possibility of predicting, i.e. describing throughout space and time, the history of the cognitive mechanism of an agent A. A's cognitive mechanism is the subject of prediction in the upper part of table 9.2. There are two situations considered. The last line of the table is simply to contrast both of these situations with the standard situation of predicting the rest of the physical world.

We considered first the case where nobody was going to interfere

Table 9.2   The logical status for the outside observer, O, and for the agent, A, of predictions of the future state of A's cognitive mechanism and of the rest of the physical world

Subject of prediction	Condition of prediction	Best attainable prediction is	Logical status of prediction
	No interference with A	CM(t): accurate UNLESS believed-by-A	Relativistic (locally valid) Untruthful-for-A (has U-claim *only* on Os)
A's CM	Interference with A	$CM_1(t)$:accurate IFF believed-by-A	Relativistic (locally valid) Optional-for-A (has *no* U-claim on A)
Physical world excluding CMs (e.g. time of sunset)	Irrelevant	Accurate and unconditionally beliefworthy-by-all	Universally valid (has U-claim on *all*)

CM denotes the agent's cognitive mechanism; CM(t) its predicted state at time t; U means unconditional; IFF means if and only if.

with A, but observations were going to be made by a spectator, someone who was not in dialogue with A. Such a one, O, the non-participant observer, is able to come up with a predictive description CM(t) where t is future time, showing how CM will develop and act throughout future time; but what we found was of course that since A's believing anything necessarily, by definition, requires A's cognitive mechanism to change, CM(t) could be accurate only if *not* believed by A. So the best attainable prediction by the observer O is a prediction which will be accurate *unless* believed by A.

This means, of course, that its claim, its logical status, is relativistic. That is to say, you have to ask from which standpoint you are talking. From O's standpoint CM(t) is accurate. From A's standpoint CM(t) is untruthful (we suggested that as a good word for it). It is untruthful because an A who believed it would believe a mistake, because A's believing it would make it out of date and as a result it has no claim to A's assent. The abbreviation U-claim stands for unconditional claim, and what we are saying is that CM(t) has an unconditional claim only on detached observers – those who are related as non-participants to the events in question – and not a U-claim on A, whether A knows it or not. A (in this first situation) does *not* know it, but nevertheless CM(t) cannot claim to be what A would be correct to believe and mistaken to disbelieve if only he knew it.

Then we went on to the second possible situation, where we imagined someone inventing a description $CM_1(t)$ which would become correct provided that A believed it. So in dialogue with A, O was going to produce $CM_1(t)$: $CM_1(t)$ *would* then be something which A would be correct to believe, as it wouldn't become false if believed by A. But on the other hand, $CM_1(t)$ is accurate if and only if believed by A (the iff is the logician's shorthand for 'if and only if'). What follows from that is not a question of whether or not A will believe it: that's not the point. The point is that logically it has no unconditional claim on A because A would be equally correct to disbelieve it. A would be equally correct to disbelieve $CM_1(t)$ because an A disbelieving $CM_1(t)$ would be disbelieving something that was not accurate: $CM_1(t)$ is accurate if and only if believed by A.

So in dialogue with A, the hapless observer O has to admit that there does not exist a specification of A's immediate future with an unconditional claim to A's assent. With the 'doctored' second prediction we're still in a relativistic situation; we're still in a situation where a detached observer would be correct to believe one thing, but A is correct to believe something else.

Having a part in determining the future and the scope of that part are as much a reality and a question of fact as having a field of action. The notion that either physical determinism or divine sovereignty could absolve us from our responsibility in doing so is, I think, an illusion based on the neglect of some necessary distinctions in logic.

10

Where Do Ideas Come From?

As in the previous chapter, I have three rather different questions to take up under this title, but again I hope the connection between them will become clear:

1 What part do random processes play in brain strategy?
2 How do such events look in a theistic perspective?
3 Conversely, what bearing has the analysis we have been carrying through, of what it means to be a human person, on our use of human personal language to refer to God?

What part do random processes play in the brain?

In chapter 9 we made the assumption of determinism, so as to give the sceptic – the one who would deny human responsibility – all that he could hope for, but I stressed at the time that there wasn't strong evidence for it in the brain. As I am sure you have gathered, both experiment and theory suggest that a significant part *is* played in the human brain by processes that the physicist would classify as random. So what I want to do now is to ask a question from the other direction. If it is not realistic to picture human brain processes as deterministic, what part do random processes play?

Notions of randomness

Lawful randomness

This requires us to make a distinction between two notions of a random process. We often refer to processes as random – shuffling a deck of cards, for example – when we mean that the process is too complex for us to follow predictively through the chain-mesh of cause and effect. Now I freely grant that if someone is shuffling cards, it would be a very difficult business actually to measure, let alone follow through, the causal implications of the hand movements and so forth. Nevertheless, the notion here is not that there is an absence of law governing what is going on, but simply that application of physical law to the situation is so complex that we give up and we say, for practical purposes, that this is 'unpredictable'. [*We say this of many situations – sandstorms, avalanches, even the fall of a leaf.*]

Nowadays there is a branch of mathematics which rejoices in the name of 'deterministic chaos' and that phrase usefully emphasizes the two facets of this. There are situations, such as the classical model of molecules in a glass of water, where billions of molecules are batting about in the void. All are obeying – in classical physics anyway – strict physical laws, but behaving chaotically, in the sense that tiny changes might determine whether or not one molecule collides with another, or grazes it and so forth. As a result, things get progressively more unpredictable as time goes on, on the basis of any limited fraction of information from which you start. Yet the events, however unpredictable in practice, are determinate.

So one notion of randomness is that you have what is called 'deterministic chaos', but not an absence of law. [*The essential aspect of deterministic chaos is that near-identical initial conditions diverge exponentially in time. Vast numbers of particles or huge complexity are not of the essence. A nice demonstration, on sale in toy shops, is a magnetic pendulum which moves under gravity in the field of several fixed magnets. Because the magnetic bob can turn on its string, the effective 'landscape' of magnetic ridges and valleys in which it moves is constantly shifting. The pendulum bounces around irregularly and unrepeatably until it runs out of energy.*]

'Heisenberg' randomness: lawless

The second notion of randomness arises from 'modern' or twentieth century physics where we abandon officially the idea of a uniquely determinative physical law. I am calling this 'lawless' for short, not implying that there are no predictions to be made, but accepting that such predictions can only be statistical, and that in the last analysis the behaviour of, say, two electrons that collide is not uniquely determined by the prior condition of the electrons. Now this may or may not be the case; that is not my point at present. My point is that the concept exists of *lawlessness*. It is associated with the name of Werner Heisenberg. Heisenberg randomness means a randomness which defies, even conceptually, the possibility of determination, regardless of the power of the computing process you have to cope with the complexity.

Random processes as seen from the I-story: inventive and exploratory thinking

Could random processes in either of the above senses play a sensible part in the functioning of the brain? If the brain suffered random disturbances in either sense, wouldn't this just result in the making of occasional mistakes? How could sense come out of nonsense? Superficially, of course this is a very rational objection. Insofar as we are thinking of purely deductive processes – deductive thinking and so forth – I daresay it would be hard to invent a context in which perturbation of the process by a random disturbance would be useful. But one of the things our chapter title reminds us is that, in human experience of what we call thinking, there are many aspects which are perfectly respectable intellectually, yet which are not deductive. An example is exploratory and innovative thinking, such as a scientist has to use when he is confronted with a heap of new evidence, and wonders how to make sense of it. Exploratory thinking is very different from deductive thinking as regards the potential benefits of turns of events that we might call random.

Think of it from your own standpoint for a moment: if you shut your eyes for a few moments I'll guarantee that each of you will afterwards be able to bear witness to experiences in which 'it occurred to you' that you had forgotten to turn the gas off, or that you ought to pay a bill tomorrow, or something like that. We commonly talk about things 'occurring to us'; we find ourselves 'struck by' a resemblance. These essentially passive words indicate that there is an appreciable component of our conscience experience of thinking, in which we are, if you like, sufferers, or undergoers, as well as actors, agents, generators. We might put it that our *typical* trains of thought (as distinct from our severely mathematically disciplined deductive trains of thought) have branch-points at which as far as we can tell – and as far as psychology can tell – the outcome is not determined uniquely by what went on consciously beforehand. Yet it is not normally irrational in relation to it. It may be disconnected; but it's not a mistake.

Human beings do more than carry out logically deductive operations on a fixed calculus. They invent new categories and novel hypotheses, to meet an unforeseen flux of events. They imagine unrealized situations. [*Here again, at the level of the internal workings of the brain, a degree of randomness would be beneficial, indeed essential.*]

Random processes as seen in the brain-story

From the I-story side, as we have seen, spontaneity is a common experience. On the brain-story side much activity is what the statistician would call a 'stochastic process'. (This is a better term than 'random', because to many people random suggests just 'chaos'.) A stochastic process is a process in which there is a good deal of structure, but also a certain amount of branching which is not determined uniquely by what has gone before. [*Think back to those brain cells each poised to fire when the cumulative signal from thousands of spines and other chemical conditions has attained a certain threshold.*]

The situation can be likened to a bagatelle board, a pinball machine, where a ball rolls down, bouncing off various pins. A tiny difference in the ball's trajectory can make a difference in the angle of rebound which in turn might determine whether there was a hit or a miss. So this is a process in which there is a good deal of randomness and yet it is a process which has a certain amount of law-abidingness to it: the skilled can get the ball roughly where they want it.

Furthermore – to adapt the illustration to make it a little more relevant to the brain – imagine such a bagatelle board in which the sloping surface is grooved, and the grooves themselves can be deepened, or filled up, according to what has happened. Imagine, that is, that the surface is plastic, that the balls that are successful are able to deepen their grooves, and that the balls that are unsuccessful send a signal back which causes their grooves to be filled up. That gives you a picture of a process which is stochastic but in which there can be a very strongly structured element. There can be a combination of *discipline and spontaneity*. The brain does appear indeed to embody stochastic processes of that sort. In such a system, a random shake-up, even a completely random shake-up (suppose you jolt the board), merely gives the system a chance to explore new paths. The new paths are not necessarily chaotic, but they are paths that would not have been visited, had the exploration gone on without the random jolt. So even random jolts can have merit.

[*The 1949 paper, mentioned in chapter 8, considered how random noise, introduced in the right degree at the various places in a digital–analogue mechanism, would lead to the exploration of new paths and hence the discovery of new facts about the field of action:*] If a 'vulgar error' is committed, the latter will normally be followed by a quite logical sequence, and a few cycles of feedback can enable the machine to detect and rectify the error unless the bias on the element responsible is unduly large. On the other hand, during these cycles information on the *reaction of the field to the error* has been gathered, and will therefore count as data in new logical sequences. The future course of the machine cannot be the same as if the error had not occurred (unless the information store is deliberately cleared).

[*Randomness in the part of the mechanism which selects stored information could be particularly interesting.*] The effect of a limited amount of noise here will be occasionally to allow entry to the machine's logical mill of stored information not apparently relevant to the current logical process. Doubtless this information will normally in fact be irrelevant, in the sense that it will lead to no alteration in activity; but if it is allowed, by the design of the machine, to appear even once in its output, its effect on the external field may be of great interest. [*Obviously too much noise in relation to other things going on in the machine is going to lead to chaos. The two ratios discussed in chapter 8 give us a way of specifying the amount of noise which is tolerable or advantageous when injected into the system.*]

Without begging any questions, it is interesting to compare the process with what we call 'getting an idea'. Many of the 'unbidden' ideas which flash into mind we are accustomed to dismiss immediately and perhaps even subconsciously as 'silly'. Occasionally, however, such a random thought starts a train of thought which 'leads somewhere', and we may then describe our idea as 'an inspiration'. The analogy in these terms is of course naive, but appears to be highly suggestive of possible concrete and precisely definable mechanisms simulating some of the functions which tend to be described as 'irrational' or 'undefinable' in mental activity (MacKay, 1949).

Organizing the trial process

To give you another example, at an even simpler level than the pinball machine, imagine that we have the problem of discovering, by pure fumbling, whether a path we want to follow requires us to turn right or to turn left, and let's imagine that it is in fact, unknown to us, a path where right turns and left turns alternate. This is the simplest example I was able to think of about 30 years ago to bring out this and I haven't since been able to think of a simpler one (see figure 10.1).

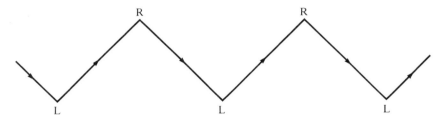

Figure 10.1   A path with alternating left and right turns.

Your problem is to find your way along the path: your brain's problem is to select from two subroutines in your brain, one to make you turn left, one right, so as to get you along the path as quickly and smoothly as possible. How could we imagine this going on? [*In chapter 3 we talked about the organizing system within our brains which runs the repertoire of possible muscular output.*] We have two 'buttons', a turn left button and a turn right button, which have to be pressed in the effector system in order to bring about an action which can be evaluated as successful in the world of the path. One possibility would be to install in the organizing system within your brain a simple coin tosser, working purely at random and coming up with a left button or a right button. On about half the occasions that would be successful, so that you would fumble your way along – but not very efficiently, because the other half of the time you would waste in being wrong.

But there is another possibility. Suppose we had a kind of 'lucky dip' in the brain: there are a lot of little tokens to be picked which, when applied, cause the left button or the right button to work. That's almost the same thing as the coin tossing, obviously. But suppose that inside this lucky dip there are connections trailing from each type of token, and these connections are of such a kind that – again purely at random – there is a finite possibility that two of the tokens, l and r, can get hooked up so that l triggers r and r triggers l alternately. These have just randomly happened to hook themselves up into little oscillators or alternators, but next time the lucky dip is used one of these ready formed oscillators may happen to get grabbed. Assuming it gets grabbed in the right phase, then having turned right, the body in question, your body, will be set up ready, conditionally ready, to turn left. So sure enough, you will succeed immediately in turning left, and next time R will turn up of course, because these are running in sequence.

If the organizing system begins with most or all thresholds fairly low, so that all kinds of sequence are possible, then after a long sequence of LRLR bends in the path the probabilities of actions which do not contribute successfully to the trial process can be steadily reduced and the others reinforced until a firm pattern of organization emerges.

Through randomly assembling in this way a little organizer of left after right and right after left, your brain has equipped you with an internal representation, in the sense we used earlier, of the alternation in the path. The path is a concrete object with right and left turns; the concept of alternation of right and left turns is an abstract concept, but it finds itself represented by the hook-up of left after right after left in this little organizing subroutine. So what we've done is to imagine a process in which factors which physically are purely random have been naturally selected, when they have occurred and were useful, in such a way as to provide the brain now with a little operational symbol for alternation of left and right in the path. Once we have got that sort of possibility, we can see how it might work at a

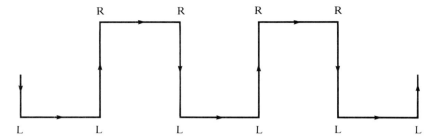

Figure 10.2   A second path sequence.

higher level. Suppose that as the path goes on, the first pattern is succeeded by a pattern of a second kind (figure 10.2) and then, after a while, the path resumes the first pattern sequence; the alternation of pattern with pattern could also be represented by a hook-up of a similar kind.

These are trivial examples, as simple as one can think of, but they illustrate the notion that processes which are physically purely random can result in *exploration* of internal representations or symbolizations of the external world. These are symbolizations which wouldn't have occurred otherwise, or at least wouldn't have been very likely to occur and wouldn't have survived long if they had. On this principle, routines which are successful in matching the world dig themselves in, their transition probabilities increasing with use. From now on the little alternator is part of the repertoire. Such an abstraction is hardly what you'd call an 'idea', although it might be an idea in a technical sense, but we can take this as an illustration of the way that an abstraction, in this case alternation, could emerge from a process which is purely random.

This then is a suggestion from the side of the brain-story that randomness could be not merely permitted, but positively valuable. Of course there is no proof that the randomness that we detect as useful in the information processes of the brain is the correlate of our experience of spontaneity and having new ideas, and I wouldn't want to insist on it dogmatically. All I would want to say is that from a scientific point of view it looks a good bet – that at least one aspect of our capacity for having fruitful new ideas may depend on the presence in our brain of stochastic processes of immense complexity. You remember those associative nets where we had tens of thousands of interconnections of variable weight modifying transition probabilities and so on. Some randomness there may well be the correlate of at least a large component of our experience of having new ideas.

It will not have escaped your notice that this is in some ways logically analogous to the sense in which the Darwinian theory of evolution, with mutation and natural selection, suggests that new species and 'improved' species (from the biological point of view) could arise out of processes where the individual ingredients were purely random. In the brain there would be good reason, from an engineering point of view, to allow random processes to operate in a context in which those which had fruitful consequences would dig themselves in, reinforce their connections, and as a result enter the internal vocabulary of the representation of the external world. They are in a very obvious sense determinants of the state of conditional readiness: having that little subroutine in your repertoire doesn't mean you are doing it; it just means that if you need it, it's there and can be used.

Development: progressive increase in dimensionality

In case you feel that this sort of thing depends too much on having things pre-fabricated, let me say that indeed if the trials were such that the probability of failure was enormously greater, or less, than the probability of success, then this would be a rather poor strategy for developing useful new ideas. The amount of information per trial is very small unless the probabilities of success and failure can be made more nearly equal. A solution is to form a kind of syndicated learning process in which at first large numbers of elements, destined eventually for independence, should be coupled together so as to reduce the diversity of response. A baby's hand and arm, for example, might not at first have each finger separately controllable, but could work clumsily as a whole. If the internal repertoire is such that the degrees of freedom (the number of independent controls) can be to some extent varied in number, you can couple controls together by statistical links with low thresholds to form something sufficiently crude that it can be tried out with a good probability of success. On this principle, if pursued to the limit, even the earliest trials could have a non-negligible chance of success (though success in a very small way).

Given this easy start, simple self-organizing subroutines can build up fairly quickly. The system starts with crude capacities, so relatively quickly it finds simple organizers to match the task in hand. As these increase in number and success, however, the system can afford to make its own task more difficult by dissolving the couplings between elements, thus enlarging its complexity of repertoire. It has been shown, mathematically, that the process of elaboration can proceed with high informational efficiency if the system keeps complexity increasing step by step with the degree of development of successful internal matching subroutines. Fully adaptive behaviour can be enormously more quickly developed than if the system started with the full repertoire to be explored. So it is not absurd to imagine that highly complex abstractions could develop – whereas if you didn't have this principle of progressive disconnection and elaboration, the chances of hitting on a highly abstract complex representation are obviously very low.

Again, this is parallel to the biological theory of evolution, where the same point is made. Hitting on the structure of the eye in one go is highly improbable, but if you can think of it – and I'm not saying that you can, but some biologists think they can – as a succession of processes in which you have progressively differentiated by stages, each of which had good probability of being reinforced, then you're in business, and the thing is not impossible.

Disciplined spontaneity

In all, we find that this picture of our own brain is developing a different aspect from the deterministic one. It has a disciplined spontaneity, whose physical roots may go deep. How deep we cannot tell – perhaps even into the atomic and sub-atomic structure of our physical embodiment. Now this is important: there is all the difference in the world between the human brain and the sort of thing a computer programmer might build as a model of such spontaneity, in which the processes which we call 'random' would be represented in a computer by looking up a table of random numbers. Looking up a table of random numbers is just following a rule and has no metaphysical interest. But appealing to the natural world to determine for you the course of your own thinking – as we all do, if I'm right, by just letting our brains run – that has an interesting significance in that the appeal depends for its outcome even on the atomic and sub-atomic structure of our physical embodiment. In this sense an essential part may be played in the generation of our ideas by events that a physicist would classify as chance.

Is there any significance for Heisenberg randomness in the brain?

You might ask whether there is room in brain events underlying mental processes for randomness of the Heisenberg variety, or whether this is all averaged out? I would say you can take two lines on this. You can certainly say (I would anyway) that most brain events involve so many million electrons, and so on, to which Heisenberg uncertainty applies, that the chances of a Heisenberg-uncertain event having a *significant* effect on most of them are virtually nil. Just as we turn light switches on and we never expect Heisenberg's principle to prevent the bulb from glowing, so it is in the nervous system.

On the other hand, there is the point rightly insisted on by Sir John Eccles, whom I quoted earlier, that when you come to something like a single synapse you are dealing with the diffusion of molecules through maybe a few dozen meshes of a membrane where Heisenberg uncertainty *could* significantly affect the probability of a molecule getting through. It is a noisy situation, with Heisenberg noise in it. Eccles has a model different from mine, where he doesn't talk about the person as embodied in the brain, but as inhabiting another world and acting on it. He is prepared to have the mind acting on these membranes, and modulating the transmission of chemicals. Now whether you like the model or not, the physics is fair enough. You can't deny that, sometimes at least, there could be events which had no causal precursor other than the Heisenberg wave-functions involved, and which therefore were – for physical purposes – lawless. If that is the case, it is still a good question whether these events are to be thought of as more significant than those that are lawful, or less. My own inclination is to say that probably they are less, rather than more significant, because they reflect less of what went on previously in the person's thinking. Although physical randomness in the brain might secure the *unpredictability* of a choice, it would seem to weaken rather than strengthen the chooser's responsibility for the outcome.

Theism

As you will realize, one of our questions in this book is what bearing the mechanistic theory of brain function has on the credibility of a religious interpretation of our human nature. Our task is not to advocate any particular religious interpretation, but rather to ask ourselves, as critically and as clearly as we can, what bearing the theory has on the credibility of a leading contender [(*i.e. traditional Biblical theism*).] While we were hammering on the theory of physical determinism, you may have wondered whether we weren't boxing ourselves into a corner, from which any meaningful contact with God – if God there be – was excluded. Now for reasons that some of you may have guessed (see chapter 9), I don't believe that even the most extreme physical determinism would have that logical consequence. But in any case, we have been seeing (as we looked at the fine detail of cell behaviour) plenty of reason to discount the strictly classically deterministic theory as essentially unrealistic. It is perhaps time to take stock and ask how our emphasis on physically random brain processes affects this same issue.

In thinking theologically about the real world of the real brain with its blend of discipline and spontaneity, a lot is going to depend on your theology of nature, and especially on your theology of chance. How would our human situation appear in the light of a theistic understanding of the physical world? Here it is of course routine, and important, to distinguish between theism and deism. The term 'theism' I will be using to refer to the idea that our world owes its being to a personal Author who is immanent in the events of our world, in the sense that if it were not for his continuing power as author, there would be no more events. I shall intend immanent not merely in the sense that he guides and pushes things around, but in the sense which would apply to a picture on a television screen – that if there were no sustaining programme, there would simply be nothing more to see. Things on the screen wouldn't obey different laws, or something like that. Without the sustaining programme the world on the screen would simply not be – there would be no more events. I am thinking of theism as the view of our world that sees it as a theatre of events with an Author whose continuing upholding power is represented by the continuing presence of the events and the objects of our world. He is in that sense immanent in our world as well as (in an important sense that will become clearer) transcendent over our world.

I say this in order to distinguish it from one (at least) variety of what is called deism, which, by contrast, sees God as an original manufacturer, a giver of being 'in the beginning' in some chronological sense, to our world. Let us say a 'constructor'; the watchmaker image is of course a famous one. As constructor he is thought of as holding off from his world, transcendent over it. If indeed he is to be thought of as active in relation to his world at all, it is by way of interference; an interference which some would pronounce theologically impossible and others theologically distasteful on the ground that he ought to have thought of it before the need arose. I mention deism only to point out that we are going to be discussing the theistic concept of God held by and large in western Christendom and indeed shared in much of its important aspects in Judaism and Islam, and not the deistic notion.

Briefly then, because it is a huge topic in itself, how does theism view the world of nature, including the world of the mysterious structures inside our heads?

The dynamic stability of the world

First, obviously, the stability of our world – which is a plain fact of experience (chairs and tables sit there, to be handled and dealt with) – is declared to be a dynamic stability. This, as you know, is in line very much, for what it is worth, with the kind of emphasis that modern physics would make. Physics would say, not that this bench is really empty space, or any such nonsense, but that the solidity and impenetrability of this bench is the fruit of coherence between a myriad of micro-events, each of which, if you were to study them with the tools of physics, would emerge as emission of photons, exchange of gluons ... I don't even know the jargon for all the latest things. The focus is all on a theatre of events. It's not a 'buzzing, blooming confusion', but it is indeed a complex theatre of events in and through which we are able to rely on the solid stability of the bench.

The coherence of the world

Secondly, the coherence of the Author's maintenance of the succession of events is the basis of natural science. Natural science is the discipline of codifying the pattern of precedent according to which we find – sometimes taking it for granted, at other times to our astonishment – that there is a coherence, a coordination between this happening and that happening, this earlier happening and that later happening, the synchrony of those happenings, or whatever. This coherence between the pattern of events is, in theism, traced directly to the coherence of the Creator's will in giving being to the succession of events. Science is a codification of the pattern of precedent according to which these events are given their being.

Scientific law

Thirdly, scientific laws describe patterns of coherence, and in that sense you can say scientific laws are purely descriptive. But we have to recognize that in the actual practice of science, scientific laws are prescriptive as well. They don't prescribe what happens, but they do prescribe the *expectations* that we are entitled to on the basis of precedent. So when we say scientific laws apply in the brain, or when we say there are some events to which scientific laws don't apply in the brain, then from a theistic standpoint we are not distinguishing between things that God has something to do with and things that God hasn't; we are distinguishing between those events to which he gives being according to a pattern of precedent, and those events – if there are any – to which He gives being without observing any particular pattern of precedent. Of course it is important to see that the whole history of natural science, from a theistic point of view, does not in the least rule out the possibility of unprecedented events. Indeed, from any point of view it is obvious (if you are tough-minded enough) that the number of thousands of years in which you have observed a particular pattern of precedent doesn't logically entitle you to say that the unprecedented will not occur.

Chance

When we turn to events without a discernible pattern (and I suppose in physics the 'Heisenberg' type of event, the explosion of radium atoms, for example, would be the standard sort of case) they may – as far as our observation goes – fall only under *statistical* laws. The best we can do is to write probabilities as to whether or not they will occur in a given period of time. Quantum physics abandons the idea of tracing micro-atomic events to precursors according to a determinate formula. It says 'if you want to predict them, hard luck!' But from a theistic standpoint, these events which are called 'random' or 'chance' are no less dependent on the creative word of the Author, the Author's sovereign fiat, than any other. If those events don't happen unless the Creator gives them their being, then He is sovereign over them, however unprecedented they may be according to causal precursors. (Quantum physics, like all physics, is of course agnostic as to whether or not there is a Creator.)

Now you must have read many discussions about events which are the product of 'pure chance – free but blind'. This was a famous phrase of Jacques Monod, the atheist. He purported to deduce from the fact that, in his theory of the origin of species, there were events which were purely random events, that 'Man at last knows that he is alone in the immensity of a universe in which he has emerged purely by chance'. In other words, Monod was trying to deduce a metaphysical conclusion that there was no purpose or meaning in the emergence of *Homo sapiens* from the technical scientific allegation (which is fair enough) that there was no causal precursor to the events in and through which *Homo sapiens* eventually developed. Now I hope it is clear that this is a complete and very revealing *non sequitur*. It is an example of wishful thinking, because in fact the coherence of events does not in the least imply that they are more dependent on the creative fiat of a divine Author than the incoherence of events that we can only classify as random. The idea 'random' is not equivalent to 'meaningless'; it simply means patternless.

If you are a theist at all, you see, your view is that the content of the Author's drama, the Author's space–time, is up to the Author. It is entirely up to Him if He wishes inhabitants of the created world to recognize some of the events as random and others as law-abiding. It is entirely for Him to say what degree of coherence there is between events. But apart from His creative fiat, none of these events will take place, whether we classify them as random or not. Random events are no less within His creative sovereignty than events which we call law-abiding.

Divine 'control'?

[The point which follows might be mistaken for a verbal quibble over the use of the word 'control', but it goes much deeper. D.M.M. is spelling out the

mental images which are and are not appropriate if an author is the creator of a world. If Shakespeare lays down his pen while writing Hamlet, *the population of Elsinore do not scamper about 'free of control'. Any such thought is ludicrously inappropriate. Independently of Shakespeare, Elsinore and all its events have no existence – and the same applies to any world held in being by a Creator who speaks and it is so.*

While personal beliefs are not strictly relevant to such a discussion, it can perhaps be mentioned that D.M.M. firmly believed in the sovereignty of God, and his aim below appears to be to strengthen *rather than weaken our conception of God's activity. He is certainly not seeking to undermine the kind of trusting reliance which is expressed by the popular phrase 'the Lord is in control'. He wrote elsewhere: 'It seems to me biblically undeniable that God as Creator is sovereign in every twist and turn of every man's daily life.' D.M.M.'s object, as I see it, is to warn us against the group of potentially misleading images implicit in words such as control, i.e. that there could be greater or less manipulation exerted; that the creation has its own independent existence; that it could, in the absence of its creator's hand on the tiller, have 'run its own course'; that only by interference can the creator affect the course of events. D.M.M. is concerned – as befits a good Calvinist! – to direct us to a stronger image free of any such deistic tendencies.*]

Now you may suppose that this leads straight to the conclusion that our divine Author *controls* all the events in His creation. Here we go back to a topic which came up in the theory of servo-systems. I argued in chapter 6 that it is inept to speak of a servo-system as controlling its own evaluator: it has its being in its evaluator. By the same token, it is inept to want to claim that we control all the processes in our brains. If the processes in our brains embody us – if we have our being as conscious agents through our embodiment in our brain processes – then of course there will be some of those processes which are the correlate of our controlling our limbs or whatever; but that doesn't mean it makes sense to say that we control those processes. We control our limbs in and through those processes: we are, if you like, embodied in, given our being in and through those processes.

The same logical point applies here: it would be inept, I suggest, to speak of the divine Author, as so conceived, as *controlling* the random events in His creation – or for that matter any of the events in His creation. Because to control is to determine form by action under evaluation (at least, that was our definition of control). To control is to act under evaluation of the action. An author is precisely not an actor in his own creation. If you write a story about John and Mary, then you are not, as author, one of the actors in the story. You determine the contents of the story, but you don't control events in the story: you give being to the whole story. Your relation as the author, although determinative in an important sense, is quite different from that of controller. A controller is a denizen of the world created, with more or less power to select and determine form, by action within the world. Authors, by contrast, don't act. They utter and it is so.

So my first point about God-talk in relation to our world is that the sovereignty of an author is not to be confused with the sovereignty of a controller. It is a sovereignty, as we shall see, but it is not that of a controller. By the same token, the idea (put out by, for example, the Archbishop of York (John Habgood), D.J. Bartholomew and others) that God doesn't control chance processes, but 'uses' them in the control of His world is, I suggest, inept, if by 'God' we are talking of the Author. If God is the Author of our space–time, then random processes are not the sort of thing that He has to 'use': He simply says, and they are. He doesn't use them to control anything else because as Author He hasn't got any controlling to do, He has merely uttering to do. He utters and it is. That's what a theistic concept of divine Authorship, I believe, means.

God-in-dialogue

You may say, doesn't theism also talk of God as pleading with men, as being disobeyed, as being frustrated and so on; surely there is plenty of talk in classical theism which justifies the idea that the sovereignty of God is not unlimited?

Here we come back to the logical point that we were trying to clarify in the previous chapter. Yes, of course, it is undeniable; and yes, there is no experience of theistic religion in which its practitioners would not bear witness to the reality of situations where they were aware of the will of God – as they would say – and went against it and were ashamed of themselves and came back for forgiveness. You wouldn't make any sense of the teaching of Jesus, unless you recognized that this was meaningful in talk about God. So how does this square with the idea of theism, that God is Author? I suggest that we take this in stages and use hyphens again.

God-in-dialogue is a concept which is personal, and it does go with concepts such as pleading, exhorting, admonishing, forgiving and many others that are familiar to us in classical theism. Theism certainly holds that dialogue-with-God can be, and is, part of the human experience, part of the I-story of created human beings. Now, you remember, we have always insisted that what we have to talk about when we want to keep our feet on the ground is what people *experience*. The I-story points: it is our best way of verbally pointing to those data of conscious experience which we would be lying to deny. There are plenty of witnesses, as we all know, down through the ages, to the claim that dialogue with God can be part of experience, part of the I-story that they would be lying to deny. So our question now is not, of course, whether it is true, but where such talk could fit in. Is this coherent with the whole perspective that brain science has been sketching? There are two kinds of objections that I'd like to look at.

What is the physical correlate of dialogue with God?

First of all, from the standpoint of physical science it could be argued that we are talking about conscious experience which the brain scientist assumes to be embodied in a physical process inside people's heads; in other words a process 'obeying physical laws', a process which ought to submit to analysis of a scientific sort, similar to that you would apply to the lungs or the heart or the kidneys. Now of course we insisted that there was an information-processing level which had to go into analysis of brain activity, but we also insisted that that didn't afford to neurons any privileges to disobey the ordinary physical laws; it simply meant that you would have missed the point of what was going on if you didn't analyse it in informational terms. We are not going to renege on that and say 'perhaps physical laws are disobeyed in the brain so as to allow dialogue with God to be possible'. No, on the contrary, if we are going to take the notion of theism seriously, what we have to ask is: what might be the correlate of the experience of dialogue-with-God?

Obviously we are speaking in the fog of our ignorance, but I think it is possible to fasten on aspects of what we do know and to recognize at least one possible answer. What has become clear in our analysis is that much of our experience, more particularly in contemplation, meditation and so on, involves stochastic branching where the precursors of the branch (down this way or that way) were not adequate determinants of the branching. Within the multi-million-fold activity in a human brain, if we could, as it were, 'magnify up' regions of activity here and there, what we would find is a stochastic process of immense complexity in which spontaneous transitions are happening all the time.

Now if – and it *is* purely 'if' from our standpoint – if it is the will of the Author of our being that some of these transitions shall have the significance of dialogue-with-Him, in the course of acts of worship, acts of penitence or meditation or whatever, then there is absolutely *nothing* that I can see in the spirit or the structure of physical science to prevent this from being a genuine experience of, if you like, engaging with the Author-of-our-being in a process which, as far as we are concerned, we undergo. As I mentioned, we even bear witness to undergoing such things as being struck by a resemblance or suddenly remembering that we'd left the gas on. 'Being struck' doesn't, from a psychological point of view, distinguish such events significantly from being struck, for example, by the realization, when you read the life of Christ, that you've got some grounds to be ashamed of yourself. Now as I say, we are only discussing the compatibility of these ideas, not their truth; but it does seem to me to be a fair claim that there is nothing whatsoever *incompatible* between the testimony of religious people down through the ages that their experience can take the significance of dialogue-with-God, and the most tough-minded of mechanistic images of what goes on in their brains as the correlate of those experiences. It needn't be a very formal act of meditation, just scratching their heads and saying: 'God, what would you like me to do now?' But their experience in thinking things through can take the significance of dialogue with the God whom they believe they have come to know.

Now at once you'll want to ask how one distinguishes this from sheer superstition? The answer is, of course, that not everything that comes into our heads is supposed, on theistic presuppositions, to be a communication from God. We're not asking if we can, as it were, baptise every stray thought that crosses our minds as a gift from God – a divine communication. What we are asking is whether, among the whole flock of events that occur to us spontaneously, there is room for the Creator to give being, sometimes, to an experience in us which is an experience of recognizing His will, seeing it more clearly, or whatever it may be.

So I would say that from a religious – and certainly from a Biblical –

point of view, the duty to be on our guard against superstition is a prime duty because we are supposed to be concerned with a God who among other things is a God of truth: a God who detests tomfoolery of all kinds. The hint which we have in the New Testament that we must 'test the spirits whether they be from God' is a good indication that there will be ingredients in the trains of thought that cross our minds which will need sifting out. It takes for granted that a sifting for those ingredients for which we can thank God – as distinct from the ingredients that are neutral or, worse still, temptations – is a matter of actual discipline. In that sense this process of being struck by ideas, some of which may genuinely be from God, is not so very different from what we were saying about the other stochastic processes; there is spontaneity, but it is disciplined spontaneity. The discipline of a realistic theology of God is meant to operate as an antidote against superstition.

What logical scope is there for dialogue with God?

Now we come to the last objection that there is room for, and this is from the standpoint of logic. People might say this sort of thing sounds as if it involves a self-contradiction, because you have just been insisting earlier that the author is not a controller and is not a participant in his own drama. No author who writes a story is a participant in the story. So what room is there for talk of God-in-dialogue? I must say that if God-talk were reduced to talk of one person on the model of the human person, then it would seem to me to be incoherent to seek to find room both for the concept of God-as-author and for the concept of God-in-dialogue.

The dimensionality of an author   Must we choose, then, between a monotheism with an unknowable God (in relation to whom 'God-in-dialogue' is meaningless) and some sort of polytheism? Very tentatively, as a layman in theology, I would suggest that the answer is no. We are talking now about a logical objection; I am not talking revealed theology but simply saying that the idea that there is a logical incoherence here is false. Let us suppose, as seems more than likely, that the Author of our space–time has more dimensions to His being than those of His creation. (It would be hard, I think, to have a coherent concept of an author whose 'dimensionality' in some sense –

whose degrees of freedom – did not transcend those of his creation.) If that is the case, then the richest possible projection of the author's being in the dimensions of his creation must leave some dimensions unprojected.

In case this sounds very abstract, think of the simple example of a house. A house has three dimensions. If you ask someone to prepare drawings of the house, the drawings have two dimensions. The richest possible projection of the house on two dimensions must leave at least one dimension unprojected. So you need more than one orthogonal projection in order to begin to do justice to all that needs to be said about the house. Now that is so commonplace as to be common sense. But it's a very important point when we come to think of beings, if beings there be, who have dimensions greater than ours, who have more to them than can be projected into the dimensions of our space–time in the image of a person. What follows is that such a being will require more than one personal projection if you are to begin to do justice to all that needs to be said about his multi-dimensional being. On those grounds it seems to me entirely open to consider that God-talk requires us to talk of more than one personal projection (if we are using the human being as our projective model). In particular, no single personal projection of the being of God could in general be adequate. This leads us to a whole family of distinctions.

The indeterminacy of dialogue with God

We talked already in chapter 9 about the importance of standpoint in defining the logical status of various descriptions and propositions. We were considering there the possibility of predicting, i.e. describing throughout space and time, the history of the cognitive mechanism of an agent, A, and we summarized the situation in table 9.2.

The points of logic made there apply even to dialogue with God. If it is the will of God that, through whatever process, He enters into dialogue with His creatures, there does not exist (this is a logical 'there does not') a complete specification of that dialogue and of its outcome which either of them in that dialogue would be unconditionally correct to believe and mistaken to disbelieve. So taking 'God-in-dialogue' as the name of a person, the person referred to is a person who does *not* know the future of the dialogue in which he engages. He does not have the kind of predictive – or, if you like, determinative –

timeless knowledge of the space–time of his creatures that the author has. A God, if there is a God who is willing to project Himself into our world as an agent in dialogue with us, is a God who knows us in dialogue as beings whose future is as yet *undetermined* until the outcome of that dialogue is mutually decided by the two participants in it.

What I have been suggesting is that the apparent logical incoherence or self-contradiction in the notion of the theistic God meeting us in dialogue is seen to be an illusion based on a neglect of the relativistic logic that applies in a situation where the Being of whom we are speaking may be *either* One in dialogue with us or One contemplating the whole of our space–time as its Author. If we are speaking of the personal projection of the being of God in which, as author, He contemplates His space–time, then of course the natural description would be what you find, for example, in the New Testament; that He is the one 'according to whose determinate counsel and foreknowledge'[1] all things come to pass. But if we speak of Him as God-in-dialogue, as one who has projected himself into his drama, in dialogue with his human creatures, then of that Person it is incoherent to predicate the kinds of knowledge which make abundant sense predicated of the other.

[*It should be clear that in all the above D.M.M. does not consider himself to be developing theology but pointing out that a purely technical analysis of the logic of dialogue and of an author's relationship to his creation leads to intriguing convergence with the traditional doctrine of the multi-personhood of God (the Trinity), which many people have felt to be a stumbling block of an arbitrary kind. The force of the hyphens should not be overlooked: D.M.M.'s point is an operational and logical one about the different relationships that are possible with an author who allows himself to be an author-knowable-by-his-creatures. As he says elsewhere: 'my intention is not – Heaven forbid! – to present a theory of the nature of God, but only to point out that the need to recognize more than one Person in the Godhead is logically implicit in the notion of God as a Creator who interacts with his creation.*[2]]

The will of God

This implies an essential distinction between at least two concepts of the 'will of God'. Insofar as we speak of God as personal and as having a will, we imply, of course, criteria of evaluation. But the criteria of evaluation expressed by an author in saying 'let there be', and the criteria expressed by saying 'thou shalt' and 'thou shalt not' in dialogue, are logically quite distinct concepts. An author's will cannot be defeated; an interlocutor's will can be. It isn't enough, I think, simply to classify – as classical theology has – the will of God into the 'hidden' will and the 'revealed' will, as if they were all part of one thing, but with, as it were, a hand covering part of the page. The whole concept is different because the personal projection is different. I can't say – and I'm not sure whether it would be meaningful to say – whether the projections are orthogonal, or what; but at any rate they are such that the relationship between the two is relativistic, and what can be said about the one would be incoherent from the standpoint of the other.

Finally, let me insist that multiplicity of personal projections of the being of God is not incompatible with the unity of His being. In particular, if the Author of our drama has made Himself also a participant, then distinctions of the sort that we find in Christian theism between the persons of the Father, the Son and the Spirit are very much of the kind that we would expect to be needed to do justice to the strange reality that we have all to reckon with. But to pursue this now would take me well beyond my brief.

Notes

1 The Apostle Peter as reported in Acts 2:23.
2 For a fuller treatment see MacKay (1978, 1988).

11

Knowing More than We Can Tell

I have been insisting from time to time as we talked about the relation between what we called the I-story and the O-story that the I-story that we can all *tell in words* about our conscious experience is limited in its accuracy. Although we are well able to perform the operations that lead to our saying things like 'I recognized his voice', 'I suspected that he was not telling the whole truth' or 'I realized I was going to be seasick', there is no suggestion that all that we consciously experience can be put accurately *into words*.

In our 'I-story' of table 1.1 the phrases 'I like such and such, I feel such and such a sensation, I see such and such, I believe so and so' are verbal pointers to data which we would be lying to deny, but data which make sometimes a greater demand on our verbal capacity than we have skill to meet. It would be quite unwarranted to claim that we have a complete verbal account in a I-story to do justice to the facts, all the facts, of our conscious experiences. Not all the data of conscious experience are necessarily verbalizable.

This is an emphasis which is found of course in many philosophers. Even the early Wittgenstein – who had the name of being very hard-nosed and went in for what was called atomistic logic (which could be rather easily computerized as it happens) – in the *Tractatus Logico-Philosophicus* says at one point: 'there are indeed things that cannot be put into words. They make themselves manifest.' In a letter to Engelmann he says of a poem by Uhland that it 'is really magnificent. And this is how it is: if only you do not try to utter what is unutterable then nothing gets lost. But the unutterable will be – unutterably – *contained* in what has been uttered!'[1]

If you want a more recent exponent of a somewhat similar line of thought, Michael Polanyi is well known for his many writings on the subject of what he called 'tacit knowing'. In fact the phrase 'we know more than we can tell' is one that he continually reiterated. On the basis of this he liked to express doubts as to whether the process of human thinking and conscious experience in general could be mechanized since, as far as he could see, in order to mechanize anything you had to have an explicit specification of it and tacit knowledge was by definition something that you couldn't make explicit.

Embodiment of 'tacit' knowledge

Now I think that there are a lot of technical points that could be taken up here if we had more space. Let me just make one or two points about this question as to whether tacit knowledge must be beyond the possibility of mechanizing, or conversely whether any individual with tacit knowledge could not be regarded as embodied in a mechanism.

A first point is that taking tacit knowledge to be that knowledge which is possessed but cannot be expressed in words, then if we credit (non-human) animals with knowledge at all, *all* their knowledge is tacit. There doesn't, therefore, seem to me to be an exciting gradation of higher to lower as between tacit and explicit knowledge, or evidence that tacit knowledge is higher. If anything, the case seems to be the other way round. This gets some of the steam pressure out of the idea. Tacit knowledge is not necessarily something 'higher', in the scale of comparative biology at least, than explicit knowledge; it is what we share with the other animals. An animal that knows its way through the forest to its nest, or is able to recognize a predator, has knowledge which it can't put into words. And I think it would be very odd to suggest, on those grounds, that that knowledge could not be mechanically embodied in the animal's brain. On the contrary, it is perhaps easier to envisage how that could be embodied than some propositional knowledge.

Secondly, several times in the course of this book, in looking at the brain as a mechanism, we have reached the stage where it was quite clear that much of the information that mattered and that concretely represented important facts about the world might be represented implicitly rather than explicitly. Implicitly, in the sense in which our motor car steering wheel provided an implicit representation of the curvature of the drive up which it had just been driven. The angle of the wheel with respect to the goal of keeping the curvature is a representation, but it is not of course an explicit verbal representation and it would not be a representation at all in a system that did not have the goal of following the drive.

Perhaps I should leave the matter there. I don't think it is a terribly important point but it is one that has been made by people like Polanyi and I feel that it was perhaps unduly negative. The point, Polanyi's point, that tacit knowledge is not mechanizable is true only in the sense that presumably you wouldn't know how to write an explicit digital computer program to embody tacit knowledge because by definition you haven't got the explicit entries for the program. In general it is not necessary, I think, to conclude that there can't be a mechanistic basis for tacit knowing as much as for explicit knowing.

Somebody might point out that the things that animals cannot talk about are not inherently inexpressible, for we *can* talk about the things that animals cannot talk about. I do agree, and it is something that I have often argued: the fact that knowledge is tacit in an animal does not prevent *us* from giving explicit expression to those facts of which the animal is aware. So that we could write a computer program for a model of the animal to behave in a similar way with respect to what the animal knows – but not I think with respect to the animal's *knowing it*, if you will take the distinction. Your 'spotting-something-as-a-predator' is an event in you which depends on parallel processing and it is very much an open question whether anyone can write a computer program (i.e. according to explicit rules) that will process the information in the same way. Computer people are having great trouble trying to develop programs to do just that. Maybe they will manage it; but it is going to be in the end a very clumsy, circuitous alternative to the neat simple associative parallel processing drill that goes on in the animal. So I think one does want to distinguish between saying I can write an explicit specification program for the state of affairs that the animal is aware of, and saying I can write a model for the animal's experience of tacit-knowing (that being an experience).

Rational–irrational?

The point I should like to move on to is that I think we should clear from our minds any idea that the difference between this kind of knowledge – the 'knowledge of the ineffable' as Wittgenstein is translated as calling it, or 'tacit knowledge' as Polanyi would call it – and discursive knowledge, which you can express precisely in words, is that the one is 'irrational' and the other is 'rational'. There is a tendency for people to use words loosely and to imply that philosophers who emphasize the ineffable, for example, or the tacit aspect of knowing are 'soft' as opposed to those dealing with 'hard' knowledge which is the explicitly expressible. The idea is conveyed that the one requires and displays low intellectual standards, the other high intellectual standards.

Parallel processing

Integrating the clues

I would suggest that the contrast here is one which we have met in our thinking about the processing of information in the brain. When we say, to take an often cited illustration of tacit knowledge, 'of course I know how to recognize my mother's face, or her photograph, but I couldn't tell you in *words*', we are not in the least implying that there are not *standards* by which we would determine whether a photograph was an authentic likeness rather than a bogus one. We are not in the least implying that there is something vague and woolly about the process as opposed to recognizing the logical structure of a syllogism, or whether triangles are congruent, or something of that sort.

I believe that we are engaged in parallel information processing when we are doing things like recognizing faces, or perceiving the significance of a social situation, or things in that general category which we would find it very hard to spell out in words. This involves parallel information processing, in contrast to the sort of processing that is involved in, shall we say, following through a syllogistic argument. We have seen in the course of our run through brain science that there are strong grounds for recognizing both processes as having their part to play in brain activity.

By way of illustration let us return to the picture of the Dalmatian dog (figure 5.4). Processing this in the brain is almost certainly a highly parallel operation in which dozens of different items come in and contribute their weight (in some presumably associative network) to the triggering of a conditional readiness to reckon with a dog on a leafy pavement with his muzzle pointing to the ground over at the left of the picture. Now the point about this is that almost any feature – in fact, I suspect, any one feature of that picture – could be deleted without preventing you from recognizing that there is a dog there. So, in a sense, parallel processing *is* tolerant of a great deal of 'sloppiness', and I think it is this which leads some people to associate it with sloppy thinking. The reason is, of course, that the situation is what the information engineer would call a highly redundant one. In other words there are *many* clues which point in rather similar directions – which stir up conditional readinesses of a rather similar sort. This situation then, involving parallel processing, is typical of those in which we would be hard put to it to say just what it is about any one feature which contributes to our conviction that we are looking at a dog; certainly we wouldn't be able to identify one crucial feature.

Seeing through the irrelevancies

Furthermore we encounter situations calling for the parallel processing of many clues in a redundant environment where we may have to *ignore* certain features. Plate 22 shows two photographs which you may recognize as being of Albert Einstein represented by a mosaic of little squares each of uniform greyness. The likeness is not at first very recognizable, but if you deliberately defocus your eyes you will see that the face becomes *more* recognizable rather than less. Why is this? The reason is that the edges of the mosaic tiles have inserted a lot of information of a discrete kind as to the luminances and contours. This fine detail has nothing to do with Einstein's detailed appearance and in that sense these contours are spurious; but the presence of these squares triggers responses – presumably from those Hubel–Wiesel cells that we looked at in chapter 2. These signals from the Hubel–Wiesel cells make demands which are irrelevant to the conditional readiness that is meant to be elicited by the picture as a picture

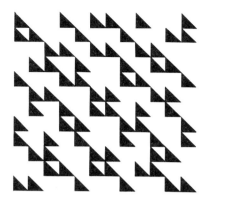 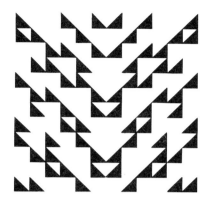

Figure 11.1   Gross pattern and fine detail. If the eyes are de-focused it will be seen that these two patterns have an identical layout: both are symmetrical about the vertical midline. The sole difference between them is that the triangular pattern elements are reversed to the right of the midline.

of Einstein. [*When, by defocusing, we reduce somewhat the weight of this distracting information, our system is able among the residue to discover a match in the recollected appearance of Einstein.*] This, then, is a situation where parallel processing or, if you like, Gestalt perception in the psychologist's sense, requires the system to set aside information that is irrelevant.

Figure 11.1 is another illustration of the same point. On the right you see a figure which has clear symmetry about the vertical midline, and on the left you see a pattern which appears to have symmetry about a diagonal. But defocus your eyes sufficiently and you see that the *gross* structure is the same in the pictures and the left is symmetrical about the midline as much as the right. Both pictures, if you pay attention only to the gross detail, are symmetrical about the vertical midline. Whereas if we insist on supplying your visual system with the fine detail then you lose that perception and perceive the left hand picture as symmetrical about an oblique diagonal.

A mode of grasping realities

These examples show that our nervous system is well equipped for a mode of perception involving the parallel convergence of data, none of which need be individually crucial, but which can be – individually – either helpful or unhelpful towards the perception of what is actually there to be reckoned with. And this is really the point: the temptation to think that this is all 'soft' or 'irrational' (there are various rude words for it) sets aside the factual question of whether there *is* indeed something there to be reckoned with. In the case of our Dalmatian the person who took the photo can assure you that he has taken great pains to ensure that there really is something there to be reckoned with whether you managed to spot it or not. And yet, although there is something to be reckoned with, discursive serial itemization is not the way to see what is to be reckoned with and recognize it.

Right brain–left brain: distinctive styles?

When we talked about the 'divided brain' and the left hemisphere's propensities versus the right hemisphere's propensities, I mentioned that, at least from the clinical evidence, there is a suggestion that our right brain is better at the recognition of Gestalts, at the recognition of overall patterns, whereas our left brain is more specialized for handling speech. The left brain is thought to be better at handling discursive formal logical structures in general, in the sense at least that people who have damage to the left brain lose this ability more than those with damage to the right. But I think that to call these two modes of knowing (i.e. the explicit and the tacit) 'left brain knowing' and 'right brain knowing', as some popular literature does, is potentially misleading. It seems to suggest that the body has somehow perversely set up two rival organizations, and it is very strange that one of them is in the left brain and the other is in the right.

If, however, we take the hint that knowing in lower animals is by definition tacit knowing – it is all they have, poor things – I think we can look at it rather differently. Our brain has the normal Gestalt perception, the parallel associative processing, which it would have had as a member of the set of animal brains. Our brains differ from those of lower animals, among other respects, in having developed, over and above this Gestalt perception, an additional skill. This, which has been developed more particularly in one hemisphere, is the skill of symbolic representation in abstract terms. This can be linked with the use of words and give us our capacity for explicit, verbally describable knowledge of our world. Language-like processing, serial deductive processing, is a special case. The normal biological process is probably the one of parallel processing, involving tacit knowledge – the sort of thing that the serial skill can get in the way of, in the left half brain.

Distributed processing

The likely physical substrate of this tacit knowing is a tangle of interconnections between nerve cells of the general kind we saw in the early chapters of this book. The contact points at the spines up and down the shafts of the nerve cells are believed to be *adjustable* on the basis of the ongoing experience of the organism – and in particular on the basis of the degree to which activity in the receiving cell was or was not associated with activity in the transmitting cell, the cell that is making the contact.

On this basis, then, we have to assume that much of this convergent parallel processing in our brains is distributed widely over the neural net. It is not that one cell does one local calculation. It is rather that within a tangle of nerve cells whose width we do not know (it may be many hundreds of cells or thousands of cells wide) the distribution of the strengths of the couplings at the junctions represents the conditional probability of reckoning with the entity recognized. Of course this distributed activity has to reach a certain threshold for the entity to be recognized. But my point is that the physical condition which determines whether or not it is likely to be recognized is the condition of a whole network and not of a local spot.

This means, firstly, that it would be very difficult for the engineer to pin down one or two crucial features of the structure and say that they were the necessary and sufficient conditions of this readiness. But, secondly, the enormous biological advantage is that since the physical substrate of tacit knowledge is widely distributed, it is also considerably less vulnerable to local damage. Local damage in one single nerve cell in such a net might make no difference to the capacity of the system to respond appropriately to the input (the Dalmatian dog's picture or whatever it is).

In case you feel that this point which I have drawn from visual examples is a 'one off' situation having no analogies elsewhere, I should perhaps mention that this is one example of a problem which has been thought of quite a lot in relation to linguistics. It has a practical aspect in that, for example, a well-designed human language is a language which, in spite of the fact that it uses logical structure and can be dealt with serially, typically uses redundancy in the same sense. That is to say, in the course of any conversation we use words many of which in a given sentence were already guessable from the context. In the course of my remarks in this chapter I will be saying essentially the same thing in many different ways. This feature – which the engineer calls redundancy – makes human language, in spite of its serial structure, much less vulnerable to local damage than it otherwise would be. We all know that misprints in newspapers, if not too frequent, can be spotted and mentally corrected almost without trouble. Why? Because the individual letter in that word has contributed to the total information pattern such a small amount of independent information that the redundancy – the probability of the couplings to all the other letters – allows us to ride over it. The same principle, incidentally, makes English a worthwhile language in which to design crossword puzzles. If it were not for the fact that the redundancy falls in the right range, crosswords would be either too difficult or trivially easy.

We can take another example from a different field: you have heard no doubt about holography – the way in which it is possible to spread the information from a pictorial scene over a photographic plate according to a principle which allows you to use any half or any quarter of the photographic plate and regenerate the whole image. Again redundancy is used to allow the processing in parallel of many clues, each of which has a very tiny contribution to make and could be lost without trouble.

We are familiar, then, in information technology and information theory, with many different situations, of which the human brain is one, where very concrete and definite information may be widely distributed. It is distributed in a form which makes its distribution vague – so vague that you can allow parts of it to drop out without disadvantage – and hard to pin down (because pinning down is localizing and localizing is precisely what you don't want to do). What you want to do is to direct attention to the coherence over different parts of the total structure. This is a coherence, statistical or otherwise, of the many different items of information – think again of the Dalmatian dog. Charges of 'vagueness', then, while technically supportable in a limited sense would totally miss the point, which is that the mode of parallel processing, by contrast with the mode of serial processing, has to be vague and prides itself on its ability to tolerate a certain kind of vagueness.

Note also the way in which, in our brains, our tacit knowledge, as represented by all this parallel structure, will be dependent on particular microscopical details and indeed perhaps sub-microscopical details of the actual matter of our brains. I stress this again of course by contrast with the program in a digital computer where you write ones and zeros to represent the truth or falsehood of propositions and there's an end of it. It is all black and white, very clear, very precise and every consequence can be deduced. But in the case of parallel processing on this stochastic basis, the microphysical details of the actual matter in your brain may be significant contributors to the content of your tacit knowledge.

Internal experimentation

The exercise of the knowledge we possess tacitly, the actual rational *use* of our tacit knowledge, requires at the physical level a continual succession of what I called in earlier chapters *appeals to local physical reality*. By this I mean internal experiments conducted in the brain – in the way in which you could call the rolling of a ball down a bagatelle board a physical experiment, to see where it is going to land at the end. These appeals to reality then, in the vast experimental theatre of the brain's associative networks, have outcomes which play an essential part in shaping both the course and the character of our embodied agency. In short, for us as embodied persons (by contrast with digital computers) matter *matters*. We have to have a respect for the physical structure of our embodiment which we wouldn't need to have if we were thinking in terms of a general purpose computer.

This raises one further point. In an associative mechanism on the stochastic lines that we were looking at in the last chapter, even the speculative trial running of ideas can be expected in general to change significantly the relative probabilities of future spontaneous transitions in given conditions. To be embodied in such a mechanism – if we are – means that even speculative questioning is not a neutral activity, but can play a significant part, willy-nilly, in determining what is likely to 'occur' to the questioner spontaneously during the whole of his future life. The moral for the philosopher may be worth pondering!

Accessing tacit knowledge

As I have already indicated, the drawing on your store of tacit knowledge – the realization of tacit knowledge – involves, essentially, a cooperative process among thousands or perhaps millions of elements in the brain. If you want an image for this you can think of the way the insertion of a Yale key in a lock makes, as it were, a test of the match between the state of the lock and the state of the key. The Yale key has only a few notches on it; but think of a Yale key with thousands or millions of notches, and think of it inserted into a correspondingly complex lock, then the business of extracting information from the system involves, in a sense, a matching of the state of all the tumblers to the grooves on the key. A Yale key is a very limited illustration because it has only one function – open or not open – but if you think of something which is like a Yale key but has the function of setting up many alternative conditional readinesses according to the configuration of tumblers on which it impinges, then you have something a bit closer to the idea of extracting the information that is implicit in our brains in given situations.

Of course, by the same token, tacit knowledge is hard, or can be hard, to share with other people. Just as your front door key matches only your front door lock and not anybody else's, so the chances are that nobody else's 'tumblers' in their brain, metaphorically speaking, will match precisely the key that you use in order to draw on your store of tacit knowledge. Giving people the kind of information that you have about your mother's photograph, for example, can be excruciatingly difficult. If you ask someone to draw the likeness that they have intuited from what you have tried to tell them, you may be bitterly disappointed. This whole problem of communication of tacit knowledge is obviously one that human beings have to work at more laboriously, and of course more frustratedly, than the exchange of serial, logically disciplined discourse. It is easy to think of objections at the verbal discursive level to the attempt to share such knowledge. When I was persuading you to perceive the Dalmatian, if you were having a hard time, you might easily have accused me of trying to brainwash you into seeing something that I was only 'making up'. And one could easily imagine a situation where I might have drawn a lot of smudges which neither I nor anybody else would rationally regard as a representation of a Dalmatian and I might have made the same noises, so there is scope for a certain amount of – what shall we say – charlatanry in the domain of tacit knowledge.

Cumulative perceptions of God's activity

Of course that is especially true of global overall perceptions of what life is all about. (At this point we come back to Lord Gifford's concern more directly.) Consider, for example, the grounds that can be adduced, by believers, for belief in God. Ask, for example, a Christian believer for the grounds of his belief that life is all about our relationship with our Creator, and what our Creator has done – most Christians would say – in history, to set that relationship back on a plane of harmony and effectiveness. Ask the Christian what grounds he has for this belief, and typically you will find that he will adduce considerations of widely different sorts, and if pinned down on any one of these is likely to say 'well, of course, I would qualify this as follows . . .'. Now I need not go into this in more detail because we all know how frequently arguments take that form. The philosopher Anthony Flew coined the phrase 'death by a thousand qualifications' to express his contempt for the non-viability of this kind of discourse purporting to justify, or provide grounds for, Christian belief. Flew sometimes has put it: 'there are Christians who imagine that if one weak argument is not good enough then a hundred weak arguments are bound to be better'.

Let's think coolly about this. I believe that talking that way shows a straight confusion between serial and parallel logic – between discourse appropriate to explicit knowledge and discourse appropriate to the perceptual, 'Gestalt', knowledge. The Gestalt type of knowledge gained by parallel processing can, I believe, be involved in religious knowledge. Suppose, for example, we were to take the Dalmatian again and somebody representing my friend Professor Flew were to grill you. He could as well – and with as little justification – use the contemptuous phrase 'death by a thousand qualifications' as a result of that kind of discussion. He could perfectly well have said: 'Well, if that particular spot there is a poor reason, you're not going to tell me that having a hundred equally poor reasons is going to make the case any stronger'. The cliché – which is totally question begging – is 'the case is as strong as its weakest link'. Now let's think about that: what kind of argument is as weak as its weakest link? Obviously it is a chain argument, it is a serial argument. It is only in a serial argument that it is true that the argument is as strong as its weakest link. If an argument is a parallel argument – one which involves the integration of much parallel evidence – it is simply false to say the case is as strong as its weakest link. All the links individually may be too weak to stand up – they may give a probability of less than half to the conclusion – and yet integration over the Gestalt (as in the case of our Dalmatian dog) may provide adequate grounds.

I do believe that someone may bear witness to a sense of the presence of God, for example, entirely rationally (that is to say not irrationally) even though unable to itemize specific experiences that demand in any 'open or shut' way, description as dialogue with God. As Martin Buber pointed out, dialogue in the sense of reciprocal interrelationship with another, even between human beings, can continue in total silence between the two parties. By dialogue we are not necessarily talking about talking *at* one another. There is a difference in other words between the experience of recognizing-the-presence-of-God and 'experiences' in the sense of identifiable events which seemed strange and which in some sense demanded God-talk. On the other hand that's not to say that people can bear witness to experiential grounds for belief in God *without* pointing to experience. Always we are back to the question: is there anything in the facts to which the I-story seeks to bear witness which, taken as a Gestalt, demands or justifies God-talk? The facts of experience are the starting point. We are not simply asking whether it would be nice to import this sort of talk – without any basis in the facts of experience to which the I-story bears witness.

I emphasize this because I think we are again in an area where we must ask what the difference is between a perception – a Gestalt parallel perception of a reality – and wishful thinking? Wishful thinking, I think, is definable as analogous to the imposing of meaning arbitrarily and baselessly on a random blot pattern. It would have its parallel in the arbitrary decision to go in for God-talk *without* anything in conscious experience – not even the Gestalt awareness of the presence of God – to point to as something that the agent could not honestly set aside. If we look (purely as samples, not as grounds for belief) at the kind of testimony offered by writers of the Bible, we find a good deal that is analogous to what we have been saying about perception in general. We find a welter of images of God, some of them very different, some of them apparently conflicting. And the question is: are we here dealing with a rag-bag in which you pick and choose what you like? Or are we dealing with the kind of evidence which, organized appropriately, *coheres* so as to bring out, in a parallel processing operation, some kind of coherent perception of One who is to be reckoned with – as the religious traditions claim?

A fuller percept in a situation of multiple dimensionality

I think there is a useful hint to be gleaned here from yet another field of perception, namely the perception of additional dimensions. I invite you to do the experiment of holding out in a straight line before your nose your thumb and your forefinger. If you close your left eye you will bear witness, I hope, to the fact that your finger is to the right of your thumb; close instead your right eye, and you will say that you see your finger to the left of your thumb. Verbally there is a straight contradiction: 'my finger is to the left of my thumb; my finger is to the right of my thumb'. What are you talking about? You have contradicted yourself! But of course any boot-faced logician (who insisted that there was a contradiction) would be talking through his hat because he has failed to identify for *standpoint* the two descriptions. The explicit statement would be 'from the standpoint of the left eye, or left pupil, the finger is to the left of the thumb and from the standpoint of the right eye it is to the right'. Given this, there isn't any necessary contradiction. But there isn't necessarily any very interesting perception either.

What we do in practice, however, is to open both eyes, whereupon we have a qualitatively new perception: we perceive the finger as behind the thumb. Perceiving it behind the thumb is the result of a parallel operation where the signals from the two eyes are compared for disparity (if you like for contradiction) and the nature of the contradictions gives rise to the conditional readiness to reckon with one thing as behind another. An additional dimension to the world is perceived by us as a result of allowing the appropriate information in two different channels to converge in parallel in the appropriate way.

I think the same is true with respect to many of the apparently disparate testimonies that we find in religious writers as to experience of God and the nature of God. There is the perception that God is one, for example, and yet bears partial conceptualization as the personal Author of our space–time, as the personal Rescuer of our sinful humanity, and as the personal Paraclete who is willing to indwell our conscious life, so as to bring out of our spontaneous thinking, valuing and choosing, something better than we otherwise could.

Spiritual life

Let us then, finally, consider what scope there is in the picture of our human embodiment as in a network of cells and so on for the category of 'spiritual life'. Note that we are not asking: is this a category pointing to a transcendent reality that we must all reckon with? That is a question of fact to be investigated in its own right. We are asking rather the philosophical question: is there an incompatibility between the whole notion of spiritual life and the notion of a mechanistically explicable embodiment of the sort that we have been considering? We find, for example, in Christian theology the emphasis on our being by nature 'spiritually dead' and of course this is said in the full knowledge that all of us by nature are also psychologically very much alive. The question is: what room is there – is there any room in our picture – for such talk? What might be the correlate in the brain-story for talk about somebody who had been spiritually dead coming spiritually to life?

When we were thinking about the transition from purely physical descriptions of biological tissue to discussions of the brain of a conscious agent, we appealed to an information-flow map of the organization of agency and we talked about the development of self-supervisory agency, that is to say of a level of organization where the priorities of the system themselves came under the range of control of the system. This level at which the system reached into its own controls and became the supervisor of its own priorities we considered to be necessary as the basis of the kind of behaviour that we would normally take as evidence of consciousness in the human organism. Our suggestion was that as we move from unconsciousness to consciousness there must in the brain-story be a definite transition at the technical level of the information-flow system. Personal agency comes in when cooperative self-supervisory activity starts up. If an injury abolished that, then personal agency ceases.

[*It might be asked why 'cooperativity' is mentioned here in connection with the ability to alter one's own goal states.*] Let us take first a simple physical example of cooperativity. If I hold a microphone up to a loudspeaker, then as we all know, it will set up a howl. If we ask where the howl is coming from, the answer is, oddly enough, that that is a mistaken question: there is no 'from' for it to come from. The howl has its being in what is called a mode of cooperativity – a closed sequence of things depending on things depending on things in a closed loop. There is no one element in the loop that you can blame, saying it is coming from there. Yet you don't normally say it has come from outside. You don't say it has come from anywhere. You say it has its being in the cooperativity of the system. The hypothesis that I have been exploring in earlier chapters – and it is only a hypothesis – is that the transition from unconsciousness to consciousness in us is a transition set up by the closing of a loop in our brains. It is a transition in which something like the howl in the microphone–loudspeaker system is set up in the supervisory system of our brain. It is a closed loop system, of course: part of the range of the repertoire of the internal system extends round to the criteria of evaluation of the system itself. But the system so set up is cooperative within its own priority scheme, in the sense that there isn't any link outside itself – just as with the microphone and loudspeaker. In that sense it is a self-running cooperativity.

So the question comes: can we see a possibility that spiritual life, if there is such a thing, could be *embodied in* psychological life as psychological life is embodied in physical life? You see the idea? We said the transition from merely physical life to psychological life involved the kindling into flame, metaphorically speaking, of a new mode of cooperativity – leading to the development of new psychological entities. One psychological tradition would talk in terms of 'drives' and 'motivations', concepts which would have no meaning apart from the development of this new level of organization where the entities are embodied in the physical activity – without, of course, involving any infraction of the physical laws that govern that physical activity.

Could we say that spiritual life, as theologians speak of it, is something to be thought of as embodied in psychological life as psychological life is in physical? I believe there is scope for this, but I would just like to end by pointing out some of the dis-analogies. The point is that we are already conscious agents before we receive spiritual life, and what changes in the man who has received spiritual life (if we are just going *prima facie* on the evidence of what the New Testament, for example, would say) is rather the evaluative priority scheme. So you might want to argue that the transition from being spiritually dead to being spiritually alive should be thought of as in essence no more than a change of mind – something that doesn't involve the development of a new entity. And you might well ask: why then the violent metaphor, the change from death to life?

Now I agree that it is not the only metaphor used. Jesus used the famous metaphor of being born afresh. But being born afresh is a pretty drastic transition too. I suggest that what is perhaps pointed to by these metaphors, although it isn't directly analogous to the change from unconsciousness to consciousness, is perhaps a change in the mode of cooperativity. A new kind of kindling of cooperative self-organization starts up on a principle which is at odds with the previous principle; the previous principle self-centred, the new principle God-centred. In other words, the principle of supervisory organization changes discretely if a man passes from death to life at the spiritual level.

Receiving eternal life is something that Jesus often talked about in the present tense: it isn't something only after we are dead. Receiving eternal life is represented as the consequence of allowing the Spirit of God to become a member of dialogue in the normative process of life (possibly in its planning and other affairs) but primarily and above all in the normative processes where one asks: what shall I put first, and what am I prepared to give way on if other things come in the way, and so on? And this then would be the basis of a new kind of closed chain of cooperativity in which one point of reference or one stage would be what was spoken of in the last chapter as the agency of the Spirit of God in dialogue.

That was what I had in mind in talking about a new mode of cooperativity. That God-in-dialogue becomes a participant in the cooperative process of norm setting. From a psychological point of view this would indeed be reducible, if you want to use that word, to a shift in priorities or at least to a shift in the dynamics of the priority-setting system. But presumably it would also be, from the standpoint of God-in-dialogue, a significant link between His nature and ours in that He, in dialogue with us, would be one system with us. He would be one system with us in that reciprocal relation where from now on things would be different in ways that we could not necessarily predict.

There is not time to go further into this, nor is it appropriate, but I do want to raise a question regarding the status of this 'new birth': if this *were* something to take seriously would it have to be classified as a miracle? I know that many Christians would say yes; but I would like to draw a distinction here between a miracle in the sense of a transaction in the real world in which the Author reveals his immediate personal concern and involvement in the situation, and a miracle in the popular journalist's sense of an infraction of physical law. It is not clear to me, at least, that if this transition from death to life at the spiritual level does occur in people, it need involve any breach of the pattern of precedent according to which their brains function. Sin, rebelliousness in the theological sense, I believe would be quite mis-conceived as a malfunction of the physical organism. (I think it is equally a misconception to think of it as a mere relic of our animal inheritance.) Sin is, in the theological context, the displacement of the Creator's priorities by our self-centred priorities in defiance of His. It is not obvious to me that either sin or the cure for the rebelliousness of sin – the transition to eternal life – need involve us in speculating that a brain scientist studying the brain of somebody in that condition would find the laws of brain organization broken.

Lastly, if we are trying to assess the credibility of, for example, the Christian view of our scope as agents and particularly the possibility of receiving a new kind of spiritual life, it would be a mistake to leave out of account what the same Christian theology sets before us as the cursedness of our drama. That is, I think, the shortest name for it. In other words, ours is a drama subject to frustration. It is under a curse. It is under a rubric which says in effect this is *not* the best of all possible worlds. In all kinds of ways our present embodiment is not the ideal. We will have perceptual blind spots: 'wishful-unthinking' as well as wishful-thinking can distort our perceptions in the domain of the spirit. If there is a God of truth we shall need all the help He can give us, both to look straight and to see straight, with honest eyes.

Notes

1 My attention was drawn to this quotation by the Reverend John Tallach of Aberdeen, who pointed out the kinship between this way of talking and some of the thinking of Kierkegaard about the way we change a message if we try to say it in a form alien to its nature.

12

And in the End?

On being embodied

Throughout this book we have been trying to explore relevant implications of the hypothesis that we, as conscious agents with an I-story to tell, are *embodied in* the information-processing system of our brains in something of the sense in which a triangle can be embodied on a blackboard in chalk, or an advertisement on the wall of a building in electric light bulbs, or an equation in a computer – rather than thinking of ourselves, as some would, as inhabiting a non-physical world, the world of the mind, from which each of us is supposed to interact with our brain, this indubitably mysterious structure inside our head.

I have been arguing that we should recognize an indisputable duality – a two-ness – of aspect or of standpoint. The two standpoints are the standpoint of what we called the I-story, in which in the first person we bear witness to facts of our conscious experience, and the standpoint of what we called the O-story, the brain-story, the outside observer story, from which it is possible to observe the functioning of our brains. This is a duality, certainly, but without the need to incur all the extra theoretical costs of dual*ism* – in the sense of a theory that there are two worlds.

We have seen that this duality of standpoint entails a relativity principle which exposes as illusory the often alleged antithesis or incompatibility between human responsibility on the one hand and mechanistic explanations of brain function – even deterministic ones – on the other. We have seen how even the richness of experience that we cannot put into words may have a scientifically understandable basis, dim though it is at the moment, and be no less rational for that. We have even seen hints of how we might think of the embodiment in our information systems of such mysteries as the transition from the state of spiritual death to eternal life of which the Christian religion speaks.

Death

It is now time to face a question which must have occurred to you more than once. Isn't this all tied too closely to the here and now of our physical embodiment, the structure which we have been exploring for the correlates of all this conscious experience? Isn't it too close to this particular distribution of matter for the comfort of those who would cherish the hope that this world is not the be all and end all – that we must reckon yet with a world to come? What are we to make of physical death? How detachable are we from our present embodiment? In the Gifford series of lectures the questions asked are not concerned with whether the teachings of revealed theology are *true*, but with how the credibility of different possible theological answers is affected by the mechanistic ideas which we have been exploring. Does the hypothesis of embodiment, in the form in which I have been summarizing it, rule out any hope of eternal life? Death, from the standpoint I have taken, would not of course be equated with such crude criteria as the cessation of heart beat. It would be, I suppose, definable as something like the irreversible extinction of the self-supervisory cooperative activity – which we compared to the cooperativity of a flame – within the information-flow structure of our nervous system. But if our conscious personal experience is as intimately correlated with this localized region of the physical world as we have been supposing, then death would seem to entail the disappearance from this space–time of the individual who was thus embodied.

I believe that is true. I see no reason to suppose that our embodiment is such that with the extinction of the cooperative flame of self-supervisory agency within our information-flow system there is anything left, hovering around. So far as this space–time is concerned that personal history of thinking, valuing, choosing is at an end.

Immortality?

In other words, if the view that we have been exploring were true, then there would be nothing automatic about immortality as there might be with certain thought models of a dualist kind where you picture a world of minds, and the minds are automatically immortal, but are for a time plugged-in in some mysterious un-understood way in quasi-physical interaction with a particular brain or a particular part of a particular brain. On that view the destruction of that part of the brain just means an ejector-seat operation whereby the mind or soul takes off and presumably waits for a new charge.[1] But on the view that we have been exploring, there would be nothing automatic, nothing guaranteed. And I must say that nothing known to me in brain science remotely suggests we should feel that immortality on those lines *was* guaranteed. So let us close in on the question: how intimate is our dependence on this particular embodiment? Or putting it the other way: is there any sense in which we are independent of this embodiment?

How independent are we of our embodiment?

At first sight this might seem a senseless question. Whatever our theory of the relation between brain and mind, we have come across plenty of evidence that if our brain is damaged our mind is correspondingly maimed, and if the damage is great enough we lose consciousness or die. If our conscious agency is thought of as embodied in our brain activity, it is even more obvious that we must keep our embodiment in good order by eating and drinking just enough of the right stuff, and not too much of the wrong stuff, if we want our minds to function normally. The simpler examples of embodiment that we looked at earlier – a triangle embodied in chalk on a blackboard, or an advertisement in electric lamps on the wall of a building – surely leave no doubt that the two, the embodied and its embodiment, are completely interdependent? Move the chalk lines, and you have a different triangle; change the pattern of lamps and you have a misprint or a different advertisement. But on reflection even these simple illustrations suggest some further questions. Although any change in the geometry of the triangle must mean some change in the distribution of chalk particles on the board, there are billions of alternative distributions of chalk particles all of which would embody the same triangle. You could even rub off half of them, as long as you didn't do it too unevenly, without making any geometrical difference. In the case of the advertisement, although any change in the wording would require a change in the layout of lamps, you could interchange any or all of the lamps without making a significant difference to the message advertised. Only when you messed about with too many of the letters would the thing become unreadable. Even more to the point, if you want to embody a given triangle, you have no need to use chalk: you can outline it in pencil or string or whatever comes handy. You can display the very same advertisement in ink on paper as in lamps on a board. In this sense there is a kind of interdependence between the things embodied and the things in which they are embodied. While something is embodied, it and its embodiment are closely interdependent. But the form that is embodied can be one and the same form, irrespective of the particular matter in which it is embodied.

So when we come to our own embodiment, there are quite a number of questions to be asked whose answers will have far-reaching consequences for our view of ourselves and our destiny. First and foremost we need to know which features of these simpler examples of embodiment are present in our own case and which are not. Analogies are fine as a way of helping us to see possibilities we might otherwise have overlooked or dismissed as meaningless, but the possibilities they suggest must be examined on their own merits, and cannot be defended just by appeal to the analogies that suggested them.

In our own case I think the first kind of independence is clear enough. Even if we assume that no change can take place in our conscious experience without a correlated change taking place in our physical brain activity, there are, as we saw, plenty of changes in brain activity that would make no difference to our conscious experience. Not only are there regions of the brain whose activity (as far as we know) controls processes of which we are unconscious, there are also many processes throughout the brain in which the nerve cells function as members of a cooperative team, so that even if their team activity gave rise directly to conscious experience, there could be various ways of dividing the activity among the team which would leave our conscious experience unaltered.

At a lower level this kind of 'independence' is even more obvious, since the molecules that make up our cells and other brain structures may be replaced many times in the course of life without affecting who we are. At this level our continuity despite a changing embodiment is like that of a river, which as the Greeks noted, remains the same river while its contents continually alter.

> It's a very odd thing
> just as odd as can be,
> that whatever Miss T. eats
> turns into Miss T.[2]

This may help us to sharpen our question. Granted that there are levels of analysis of our embodiment at which changes in the identity of components do not affect either the identity or the experience of the embodied individual, is there a higher level of analysis at which we can see that these changes also leave the embodiment the same?

It is here that we have found help from the ideas of information engineering. Consider, for example, a computer set up to answer questions over the telephone about the railway services. The railway timetable and the rules for responding to questions are embodied in its physical structure in a sense with which we are now familiar. The electronic hardware needs a continual flow of electricity through it, its transistors may 'age' and may occasionally need replacing, its functions may be shared over a team of elements so that one element may break down and another take over without any interruption of service. In all kinds of ways and at many levels, there will be physical changes that make no difference to it. Make no difference to it *as what?* The answer we have now learned to give is that these changes leave it unaltered as an information system – as a system in which the chain-mesh of cause and effect is one where form determines form (as distinct from the chain-mesh where energy and force determine energy and force). If, instead of looking at it as a mass of wires and things, we look at the flow of information through the computer from the buttons pressed by the telephone enquirer, through the central processor and information store and back to the screen that the enquirer uses, then we can verify that at that level nothing changes in the system when those lower-level physical changes occur. We have now found something invariant in the structure – something which is the direct correlate of its identity as a timetable guide. Make any changes that did affect this information-processing structure, and you would no longer have the same timetable guide.

In the human brain, as we have seen, there is a corresponding level of analysis at which the information-flow structure is preserved despite all the normal ongoing lower-level activity of biological repair and replacement. As an information system our embodiment is unaltered by most of the normal biological changes that we have been considering. Needless to say, I am not now talking about the physical changes in the brain that are necessary for the storage of information, the acquisition of skills and the like – those alterations that we considered in the synaptic strengths of couplings between nerve cells and so forth – since these represent the working of the information system as such. The fact that during his lifetime an individual remains the same individual despite the fact that he is continually acquiring or losing information, skills and habits, can for our present purpose be taken for granted. But now comes the key question. If a given information-flow structure is both necessary and sufficient to embody a given railway timetable guide, is a given information-flow structure sufficient, as well as necessary, to embody a particular individual? Is all that matters about your brain, all that identifies *you* as an individual, its information-flow structure?

Personal identity: replica persons

The point of this question has been dramatized by philosophers recently in terms of a number of imaginary thought experiments. Here I am afraid we are back to science fiction again! Suppose it were possible for a super-scientist to make a complete scan of every molecule of your brain and body, and to transmit the result to a 'molecular replicator' (which might be on the other side of the Atlantic or on a distant planet, according to taste). Let us suppose that it is in California. The replicator is equipped to produce a physically indistinguishable copy, molecule by molecule, of the structure necessary to embody you.

I must say that there are serious snags in this thought-experiment which I have not seen adequately discussed by the philosophers who blithely postulate it. For one thing, unless all the elements of the working brain could be assembled in working order simultaneously (rather than one after another) they could not possibly establish the pattern of parallel cooperative interaction that was going on when the imaginary brain-scan was made. This ongoing pattern we have seen to be so important in the real brain. Try to assemble it piecemeal, and the bit that you have half-assembled will already be running amok doing something cooperative that is incoherent. Metaphorically speaking, the information-bearing processes in the brain have a momentum as well as a pattern, and to start them up 'from cold' is not obviously possible even in imagination.

But setting aside such doubts for the sake of argument, the question is how we should regard the individual who comes into being, say in San Francisco, as you step out of the scanning booth in, say, Glasgow. He or she will (we may suppose) remember all that you remember, recognize and greet your friends out there as you would, and indeed be accepted by them as yourself. Which of the two then is really you? To sharpen the issue still further, suppose that the brain-and-body back in Glasgow was automatically destroyed as soon as the San Francisco replica came into being. There is now only one individual in the whole world who has your memories, your reactions, your capacity to relate personally and properly with the people you know; and that person is out in San Francisco. Some people would argue that for all practical purposes it is *you* who have been transported, 'by satellite' as it were, to San Francisco. It is called 'teletransportation' by those who adopt this view. Everyone connected with you – your spouse, your family, your employer – would doubtless find your phone calls convincing evidence that it was indeed you, the same old you, who were alive and well in California (despite the destruction of the body that went into the scanning booth in Glasgow) and in due course the wanderer would no doubt be welcomed home as you, and would believe himself or herself to be the same old you for the rest of his or her life. For a classical behaviourist in this idealized imaginary situation there would presumably be no question. Here is someone who behaves like you in all conceivable circumstances and so they would say, thumping the table when the argument was weak, it must be you. But would you, or should you, be happy to let your body be destroyed in the booth in Glasgow simply on the understanding that someone in San Francisco is going to think he or she is you for the rest of his natural life? As you can see I have my doubts, and to rub those doubts in, let us consider yet another scenario.

This time let us suppose that you were not instantly exterminated in Glasgow on completion of the replica person in San Francisco but you step out of the Glasgow scanner none the worse. And to, as it were, twist the knife in the philosophical wound, let us now suppose that the molecular replicator is not now in California, but stands alongside the scanning booth in the same room as yourself. Out of it there emerges a perfect replica of you, with (we suppose) precisely the same brain information–flow structure as at the moment of scanning of you. Which then is the real you? (Imagine that somebody introduces a whirlwind in which you are both blown around and in the end nobody looking on knows which came out of which booth.) Or is this now a silly question? Must we conclude that because both brains and bodies, at least at the first instant, embody exactly the same information-flow structure, there is no rational basis, even in principle, for considering one to embody you, and the other somebody else?

It must be admitted at the outset that there would be little hope of rationally convincing the replica person that he or she was not entitled to your name, status, property, family connections and all the rest. He or she would presumably remember (in conscious experience of remembering) as clearly as you do, all that led to your stepping into the scanning booth. The main difference would be that whereas you remember stepping out of the same booth, the replica person will presumably remember stepping out of a different booth, the replicator booth. Of course from then on, especially after you met each other, your respective informational inputs would be quite different so that even a behaviourist could recognize you as different individuals. When you met the two cognitive mechanisms would interact in that very important figure-of-eight relationship which we call dialogue. So the possibility of dialogue would immediately individuate you, even if there were no distinction before that point. The question is whether either of you could lay exclusive claim to identity with the you who first entered the scanning booth. If you had bought a car yesterday, for example, which of you now should have the right to claim it? And lest you think that a bit of decent negotiation might have a hope of settling such questions, let me ask how you would expect to cope if someone left the switch on in the replicator, so that a whole string of identical copies of you emerged from the booth, each thirsting after the same new car. No, in this context it would seem absurd to suggest that what identifies you is simply the information-flow pattern in your nervous system.

You can see now why I warned against misinterpreting our earlier analogies between the embodiment of conscious experience and the embodiment of triangles, advertisements or computer programs. In all these cases, two physically identical structures necessarily embody the very same abstract form. It makes no sense to ask: but is this triangle (or this advertisement, or this program) really the same, or only a replica? There is one and only one equation '$2+2=4$', no matter in how many calculating machines it is embodied. But our imaginary thought-experiment indicates that the same is far from true in the case of human centres of awareness. Rather it would seem that every embodiment of a human centre of awareness is a unique individual, and I can see no rational grounds for the idea that the destruction of one centre of awareness would entitle another to the identity of the first, merely on the grounds that the new one came into being at the moment of extinction of the first and was at that moment indistinguishable from it in its information-flow structure.

But, you may ask, isn't this rather like our common experience of waking up every morning as the same individual who went to bed the night before? And what if I have an accident and later wake up from a coma? In both these cases, I first cease to be a conscious centre of awareness, and later find myself once more embodied as such. How does this differ from having my embodiment totally replaced? From what you said earlier, you must agree that in sleep or coma a lot of molecular replacement must have gone on between losing consciousness and waking up.

I accept all this as fair comment. It cannot be the mere fact that the imaginary replica person's molecules are different that makes me deny that he or she is the same individual as the original. But even if we imagine that the replica booths are side by side in the same room and take the case where your original body is destroyed as soon as the replica body is functional, so that in the room there is never more than one individual with all your memories, associations and behaviour patterns, I think that there are crucial differences between this case and the case of sleep or coma. In these cases molecular replacements take place one by one so that complete temporal overlap is maintained between the initial and the final structure. For a fair illustration of such 'temporal overlap' imagine a gang of workmen hauling on a long rope, with a small fraction of the gang being continually replaced so that the team is always intact. In the case of our molecular replicator, however, the replacement is not of the elements of the original structure by a process designed to maintain *it* in being as such, but rather replacement of the original structure as a whole by another similar structure in another place. Secondly, as we noted, there is nothing to stop us from imagining the molecular replicator being used to multiply such replica persons indefinitely, in which case not even the destruction of the original could save the thought-experimenter from conceptual embarrassment if he wants to claim that one or any of the replicas was identically the original individual.

No, I think a straightforward account of what goes on in the imaginary replication is that an array of molecules embodying one particular centre of awareness (namely you) is scanned so that a set of different molecules can be assembled elsewhere into one or more similar arrays embodying other, new, centres of awareness. If the original array is destroyed, that is the end of you as a centre of awareness, however many people may be left around who look just like you, share all your memories, each claim all your privileges and no doubt wish to honour all your obligations. The scene is potentially chaotic, and the 'replica' participants would no doubt qualify as some sort of deluded psychopaths; but I see nothing in what it portrays to justify any panic abandonment of the concept of individual personal identity as, oddly enough, some philosophers have suggested.

Personal histories

What it does underline, I think, is the importance of an individual's history, his world-line throughout space and time in the definition of his identity. In relativistic physics (which we don't need to worry about in technical detail) the realistic picture of the physical universe is held to be not the ordinary three-dimensional snapshot that we might take with a camera but rather a four-dimensional picture in which time is one of the dimensions, popularly speaking, and you and I and every object in the world are represented by an extended worm-like object through time in the four-dimensional space–time. The notion of a world-line, as a more unitary representation of entities in the world, is already familiar in that context, and I am suggesting that in the case of us as conscious agents it is our world-line, our history, which must be pointed to in order to establish our identity. To try to pin down our identity to a particular brain structure at one point in time – even at the level of information processing – would be as inept as to try to tie the identity of Beethoven's Ninth Symphony to a single chord. What makes you you, as distinct from anyone else, is the unique sequence of personal acts and decisions made throughout your history. Human individuals must be viewed as entities extending through time as well as space, of which the embodiments at a given time are momentary 'cross-sections', so to speak.

The conclusion I am suggesting, then, is that even if the embodiment of your brain's information-processing structure were supposed sufficient to bring into being an individual centre of conscious agency, it could not be sufficient to ensure that the individual so embodied is you. Only a process that maintains structural continuity with your present embodiment (as in sleep or coma) can qualify as the physical basis of your continuing existence as an individual. Such of course is the normal biological process of renovation that links the you who awakes from sleep this morning with the you who lost consciousness in bed last night.

The hope of life hereafter

I have been hammering as hard as I can on a purely secular instance of the question of personal identity. But obviously in the light of the analysis we have gone through of the basis of personal identity, we shall want to ask what we are to say of the hope of eternal life, to which, for example, Christian theology refers. Is it ruled out?

If the hope of eternal life were based on an imaginary operation in which replications, on the lines we have been discussing, were carried through, then I think that there would have to be some special considerations to make it a rational hope. On the other hand, I would suggest that it is only if we forget the specifically theistic context in which the idea of eternal life is held to make sense that there is any need to worry that we are in danger of ruling it out.

What is real?

What does theism claim as to the nature of reality – all reality? What it claims is that there is only one Reality, namely God the Author, and what the Author brings into being by His creative word, His 'let there be'. For theism the world of physical reality – the succession of events in and through which we encounter what we call the physical world – is a succession of events each of which owes its being to the creative will of an Author. That is the view that theism sets as the context in which it also claims that death need not be the end of us. God, as the Author of all that is, is the final definer of the identity of all that is. He is not merely the authority in the sense of an arbitrator. He is the Giver of being to the identity of all that is.

'Whom God knew'

Theism would insist, furthermore, on the possibility of knowing God in dialogue. We found it was necessary to put hyphens in that expression so that God-in-dialogue could be recognized as a reference to a Person, where the Person referred to not only need not be, but could not be, logically the Person referred to as the Author of the space–time in which the dialogue was supposed to be taking place. The point being that God-in-dialogue knows us as persons, knows us in the intimate reciprocal interaction in which He knows us as determinants of some of our actions and part of our futures. He identifies us not merely as objects, but as persons – as persons indeed sufficiently akin to His own Personhood for us to be 'thou' to Him as He can be 'Thou' to us. This is presumably a large component of what is meant by speaking of God as 'having made man in His own image'. (In case you think that this applies only to those who respond positively to God, we should note that from the standpoint of Christian theism, as the biblical writers make abundantly clear, 'dialogue' can include pleading that is rejected as well as that which is accepted.) So in this context and only in this context, the Christian hope, as it is called, of eternal life is defined. It is defined specifically as what is referred to as 'resurrection', not just the persistence of a disembodied existence.

Disembodied existence?

I am not at all implying that the concept of disembodied existence is philosophically impossible or self-contradictory. Although I do not myself believe that the content of biblical theism demands taking seriously our persisting after death in a disembodied existence, I do not in the least want to imply that this is a self-contradictory notion.

There are those who would, as it were, 'go the line' of physical embodiment which I have been following, to the extent of saying that they would reject out of hand the concept of disembodied existence because all our conscious experience is associated with embodiment. That is true, we believe, as a matter of empirical fact here and now, but as far as my imagination goes I can see nothing self-contradictory in the imagined possibility of you or me finding ourselves with conscious experience (it does not matter of what) but that conscious experience not happening to include the experiences which we would call seeing our own body, or looking in a mirror and seeing something which covaries with our actions and so forth. It is all wild and baseless speculation – a speculative exercise in imaginary conscious experience – but it seems to me that it would be quite wrong to say that it is incoherent in the sense of involving a self-contradiction.[3]

Replicated body?

The emphasis in Christian theism, however, is on the resurrection of the body. It is the compatibility of this view with our mechanistic ideas that we are trying to assess. And you might well ask: isn't the idea of the resurrection then open to the same sort of objections as those I have been voicing to molecular replication? Now if this meant merely a reappearance in the same old space–time of a replica body, then certainly, as I said above, we'd have to do some special thinking. However, once you take seriously the claim of theism that there is nothing in our space–time apart from the creative say-so of the Author who gives being to the events in which it has its being, then I think it is clear that it would be for the Author to stipulate the identity of a resurrected body in the sense that is dimly analogous to the replicated body that we have been talking about out in California. It would still be possible for the Author to say: this individual who has come into being in California *is* really the same individual as the one who died over in Glasgow. That would be the Author's prerogative.

A new creation

If I understand it aright, however, the world of the resurrection that is envisaged by Christian theism is not to be reduced to just 'more of the same' at a later point in time. I see no basis for insisting that that is the thought model to which the Christian hope is pointing, even though a lot of metaphors are used which would fit with that. But there is also the insistence on the concept of a 'new creation'. Here we are in deep water theologically, but at least if the concept of creation is to be thought of by any analogy with creation as we ourselves understand it – as, for example, the creation of a space–time in a novel – then a new creation is not just the running on and on of events later in the original novel: it is a different novel. A new creation is a space–time in its own right. Even a human author can both meaningfully and authoritatively say that the new novel has some of the same characters in it as the old. The identity of the individuals in the new novel is for the novelist to determine. So if there is any analogy at all with the concept of a new creation by our divine Creator, what is set before us is the possibility that in a new creation the Author brings into being, precisely and identically, some of those whom He came to know in and through His participation in the old creation.

Seed and plant

The continuity, on that view, between us now and us in the resurrection, is one to which our embodiment would certainly not be dismissed as irrelevant in Christian theology. But it is expressly denied to be a continuity of replication. Remember, for example, how Paul writing in 1 Cor. 15 imagines an objector who says: 'What's all this talk about the resurrection? What sort of a body are they supposed to be provided with? Where do they get their body from?' And Paul says: 'You foolish man; when you plant a seed in the ground, you don't expect a seed to come up; you expect a shoot, a blade, which will be physically quite different.' He doesn't go into biological detail, his conceptions were no doubt different from ours. But the point he is making is that there is an element of continuity; what comes up is related to the seed that is put in, yet the plant is different in all kinds of ways. He spells out the differences in that embodiment – which he envisages in his doctrine of the resurrection – from the embodiment that we have here and now. There is certainly no need for the seed to be preserved: I take it that he is uttering an explicit warning, with his talk about the seed and the plant, that it is not going to be a re-assembly of the original body. Quite the contrary: he says – in the biology of his time – that the seed has to 'die'.

So what is set before us, which we are invited to test for credibility against our mechanistic thinking about our human nature, is denied to be a mere replication operation or mere re-assembly, but it is indeed one to which our physical embodiment here and now is not irrelevant. The point Paul is making is that since the seed determines what plant comes up, there is continuity. We, of course, would think in genetic terms, but the technicalities are not what matters. What matters is the combination of discontinuity of embodiment with a continuity sufficient to make it meaningful to use the same name, as it were, of the resurrected one. The doctrine is of the 'resurrection of the body' and not merely of the persistence of the disembodied.

We are here in a region where revealed theology is very economical with what it tells us but it would appear that in the resurrection the resurrected one is still able, for example, to look back in gratitude for something that God-in-dialogue did for him in the earlier phase of his existence in this space–time. That, it seems to me, is the way that continuity would be traced. The discontinuity in his priorities, whereby, if all has gone well, he loses the rebelliousness that plagued him even while he was a believer here, that discontinuity wouldn't be more disturbing philosophically than the discontinuity in his life here and now when he becomes a believer. Here, if not long before, you might expect me to apply my favourite motto: when short of data keep mind open and mouth shut. It is clear, I hope, that to me this is a deep mystery. I am only fumbling after what is supposed to be meant by a doctrine which I happen to accept; but accept in the sense that I hope it will become clear to me as time goes on rather than in the sense that I have judged it and found it true. But such hints as we find in biblical teaching, it seems to me, find no challenge whatsoever to their credibility from the direction of brain science.

The essential idea of 'eternal life', if I understand it aright, and whether we believe in it or not, is the integration of our normative process, here and now – of our whole priority scheme – with the priorities of the Giver of our being. If it is His will that the end of our conscious agency in our present space–time shall not be the last episode in our unfolding relationship of dialogue with Him, no precedents that are set by our present embodiment would seem to stand in His way, however surprising to us the ultimate reality may prove to be.

Stocktaking

At the end of this marathon perhaps it would be useful to take stock once more. What I have been arguing in this book is that we should abandon, for good reason, the Procrustean and physiologically unrealistic image of our cerebral embodiment as a species of rule-determined symbol manipulator, and recognize the functional significance of the brain, this mysterious structure that we carry around, as a theatre of internal physical experimentation, which bears the traces of its whole history in the conditional probabilities that, you remember, were such an important feature implicit in its physical micro-structure – those ten thousand million neurons with each their average of ten thousand interconnections. These set the multi-billion-fold matrix of conditional probabilities shaping what we are likely to do in all conceivable circumstances.

The neuroscientific working hypothesis that we are each embodied in such a mechanism, I have argued, would not entail the reducibility of all our behaviour to rule following. It would not entail any denial of our ability, by our thinking, valuing and deciding, to determine our own future. It would not imply that I could be teletransported from A to B merely by having someone program a mechanism at B to function in an identical manner to my brain. (It would not even imply that a mechanism so programmed could be guaranteed to embody any conscious experience whatever.) But it would raise no rational obstacle, I have suggested, to the possibility of eternal life, as specifically adumbrated in the Christian religion. I have further argued that mechanistic embodiment on these lines entails no denial of genuine creativity, nor of the reality and importance of tacit human knowledge, inexpressible in words.

Its main cost is that if for us there can be no coming to know without a change in the physical world, in what we called our cognitive mechanism, then, oddly enough, no complete future-tense specification of the physical world can exist (that is, of the physical world including our brains) with an unconditional claim to the assent of all cognitive agents. Instead, in the case of cognitive agency such as ours, we must be content to recognize a relativistic situation in which it is not necessarily the case that if O – our friend O, the observer – would be correct to believe P and in error to disbelieve P then everyone else would be correct to believe P and in error to disbelieve P. In particular, for an agent A contemplating a choice, the immediate future of his cognitive system is not just unknown, but logically indeterminate until he makes up his mind; indeterminate, that is, for him and those in dialogue with him even if his brain were as physically determinate as clockwork, which of course we have seen it is not. So the costs of mechanistic embodiment on the lines that we have envisaged do not include any implication that the future outcome of a choice is already inevitable for the mechanistically embodied chooser.

It will, I hope, be clear that in our whole series of discussions I have had no intention of urging a belief in mechanistic determinism or even in information-flow models of the brain. My aim has rather been to loosen up a knotted skein of improperly linked inferences, widely canvassed, in order that the hypothesis of our mechanistic embodiment may be disentangled and considered properly on its merits. There are some anti-religious propagandists who claim that mechanistic conceptions of brain function simply rule out the kind of assessment of human nature that we find in, for example, the Christian religion. I have, I hope, given some reasons in this book for regarding such claims as a vivid example of what we referred to as 'wishful-unthinking'. On the evidence that we have reviewed, I would argue that the further we probe into the mystery of our embodiment, the more the resulting picture seems to be not just compatible with a theistic understanding of our nature and destiny, but positively hospitable to it. In particular, the question whether all human brain activity has a mechanistic explanation, I would suggest, is one we can peacefully leave open for future investigation, no matter how high a view we take of the human being's power of decision and its moral and religious significance.

I will end with one last admonition from another Gifford lecturer, the Dutch historian of science, Reyer Hooykaas: 'Always remember', he likes to say, 'that natural science is not nature'. Nature is something that stands over against us to be reckoned with – something to which our science of nature is a response, framed in human categories. The subjectivist idea that nature is a human construct is abhorrent to that scientific integrity that seeks to understand in a spirit of obedience to objective fact. Our science of nature over the centuries has had its ups and downs, but if pursued in a spirit of reverent obedience it turns out to be objectively progressive. It is not all in vain. We are not cleverer than our ancestors (that is important to recognize) but we do know more. So let us always remember that brain science, in particular, is at best our current way of picturing that mysterious part of nature that is inside our heads. We must always be prepared for the likelihood that the real brain, as part of nature, may have an infinity of surprises in store for us. As Hooykaas likes to put it: 'To confuse our science of nature with any part of nature itself, is the same error as to confuse theology with divine revelation.' But of these matters Lord Gifford would have me speak elsewhere.

Notes

1 I do not find this metaphysical position philosophically self-contradictory or incoherent. I do not accuse people like Sir John Eccles or Richard Swinburne, who hold this view, of talking meaningless nonsense. I am open minded about it in the sense that I can't see any reason against it. But I also cannot see any reason for it.

2 From 'Miss T.', by Walter de la Mare.

3 This is not at all the same notion as the immortality of the soul. The notion of disembodied existence is an I-story notion, not a story that claims to be an objective set of facts about a world that a spectator could witness as filled with souls. It is a speculative exercise in imaginary conscious experience. The one is talking about the way things might be; for all we know there may be another world – a world peopled by minds. The other is talking about experiences you might have, and one of the experiences you might have is the experience of finding your self disembodied. I don't find either of these notions philosophically self-contradictory. But I object to both because I cannot see any strong grounds – in philosophy, in brain science or in revealed Christian theology – for believing in either of them.

Bibliography

Ackley, D.H., Hinton, G.E. and Sejnowski, T.J. 1985: A learning algorithm for Boltzmann machines. *Cognitive Science*, 9, 147–67.

Adrian, E.D. and Matthews, B.H.C. 1934: The Berger rhythm: potential changes from the occipital lobe in man. *Brain*, 57, 355–85.

Barlow, H.B., 1953: Summation and inhibition in the frog's retina. *Journal of Physiology*, **119**, 69–88.

Bartholomew, D.J. 1984: *God of Chance*. London: SCM Press.

Berger, H. 1929: Uber das Elektrenkephalogramm des Menschen. *Archiv für Psychiatrie und Nervenkrankheiten*, 87, 527–70.

Blasdel, G.G. and Salama, G. 1986: Voltage-sensitive dyes reveal a modular organisation in monkey striate cortex. *Nature*, 321, 579–85.

Braitenberg, V. 1977: *On the Texture of Brains for the Cybernetically Minded*. Berlin, Heidelberg, New York: Springer-Verlag.

Braitenberg, V. and Kirschfeld, K. 1968: Optische und neurale Projektionen der Umwelt auf die Ganglien im Complexauge der Fliege. *Mitt. MPG*, 3, 185–206.

Brindley, G.S. 1982: Effects of electrical stimulation of the visual cortex. *Human Neurobiology*, **1**, 281–3.

Brindley, G.S. and Lewin, W.S. 1968: The sensations produced by electrical stimulation of the visual cortex. *Journal of Physiology*, 196, 479–93.

Buber, M. 1937: *I and Thou*. Edinburgh: T. and T. Clark.

Carr, T.H. and Bacharach, V.R. 1976: Perceptual tuning and conscious attention: systems of input regulation in visual information processing. *Cognition*, 4, 281–302.

Cooper, S., Daniel, P.M. and Whitteridge, D. 1951: Afferent impulses in the oculomotor nerve, from the extrinsic eye muscles. *Journal of Physiology*, 113, 463–74.

Craik, K.J.W. 1943: *The Nature of Explanation*. Cambridge: Cambridge University Press.

Darrow, C., quoted in Dworkin, G. (ed.) 1970: *Determinism, Freewill and Moral Responsibility.* Englewood Cliffs, NJ: Prentice-Hall, 1.

Ditchburn, R.W. 1969: Eyemovements. In A.R. Meetham and R.A. Hudson (eds), *Encyclopaedia of Linguistics Information and Control.* Oxford: Pergamon.

Douglas, R.J., Martin, K.A.C. and Whitteridge, D. 1988: Selective responses of visual cortical cells do not depend on shunting inhibition. *Nature*, 332, 642–4.

Eccles, J.C. 1981: Voluntary movement. *Freiburger Universitätsblätter*, 74, 24–8.

Eccles, J.C. 1986: Do mental events cause neural events analogously to the probability fields of quantum mechanics? *Proceedings of the Royal Society London B*, 227, 411–28.

Elberling, C., Bak, C., Kofoed, B., Lebech, J. and Saermark, K. 1982: Auditory magnetic fields: source location and 'tonotopic organisation' in the right hemisphere of the human brain. *Scandinavian Audiology*, 11, 61–5.

Engelmann, P. 1967: *Letters from Ludwig Wittgenstein.* Oxford: Blackwell, 7.

Evans, E.F. 1964: Behaviour of Neurones in the Auditory Cortex. PhD Thesis, University of Birmingham.

Evans, E.F. and Whitfield, I.C. 1964: Classification of unit responses in the auditory cortex of the unanaesthetised and unrestrained cat. *Journal of Physiology*, 171, 476–93.

Fechner, G.T. 1862: *Elemente der Psychophysik.* Leipzig: Breitkopf and Härtel, 548–60.

Flew, A.G.N. 1955: Theology and falsification. In A.G.N. Flew and A. MacIntyre (eds), *New Essays in Philosophical Theology.* London: SCM Press, 97.

Flew, A.G.N. 1966: *God and Philosophy.* London: Hutchinson, 57. Also 1984: *God: A Philosophical Critique*, La Salle: Open Court, 57.

Ford, D.H., Ilari, J.I. and Schadé, J.P. 1978: *Atlas of the Human Brain.* Amsterdam, New York, Oxford: Elsevier–North Holland Biomedical Press.

Frackowiak, R.S.J. 1988: Positron emission in neurology. In C. Kennard (ed.), *Recent Advances in Clinical Neurology.* Edinburgh: Churchill Livingstone.

Fraser, J. 1908: *British Journal of Psychology*, 2, 297–320.

Gibson, J.J. 1950: *The Perception of the Visual World.* Boston: Houghton Mifflin.

Gibson, J.J. 1966: *The Senses Considered as Perceptual Systems.* Boston: Houghton Mifflin.

Gombrich, E.H. 1960: *Art and Illusion.* London: Phaidon Press.

Gregory, R.L. 1974: *Concepts and Mechanisms of Perception.* London: Duckworth.

Habgood, J. 1980: *A Working Faith.* London: Darton, Longman and Todd, 16–21.

Hammond, P. 1978: Directional tuning of complex cells in area 17 of the feline visual cortex. *Journal of Physiology*, 285, 479–91.

Hammond, P. and MacKay, D.M. 1975: Differential responses of cat visual cortical cells to textured stimuli. *Experimental Brain Research*, 22, 427–30.

Hammond, P. and MacKay, D.M. 1976: Functional differences between cat visual cortical cells revealed by use of textured stimuli. *Experimental Brain Research*, Suppl. 1, 397–402.

Hammond, P. and MacKay, D.M. 1977: Differential responsiveness of simple and complex cells in cat striate cortex to visual texture. *Experimental Brain Research*, 30, 275–96.

Hubel, D.H. and Wiesel, T. 1959: Receptive fields of single neurons in the cat's striate cortex. *Journal of Physiology*, 148, 574–91.

Hubel, D.H. and Wiesel, T. 1962: Receptive fields, binocular interaction and functional architecture in the cat's visual cortex. *Journal of Physiology*, 160, 106–54.

Hubel, D.H. and Wiesel, T.N. 1977: Functional architecture of macaque monkey visual cortex. *Proceedings of the Royal Society*, 198, 1–59.

Huxley, T.H. 1894: On the hypothesis that animals are automata, and its history. In *Methods and Results, Essays.* London: Macmillan.

Jonides, J. and Gleitman, H. 1972: A conceptual category effect in visual search: O as letter or digit. *Perception and Psychophysics*, 12, 457–60.

Jung, R. 1974: Neuropsychologie und Neurophysiologie des Kontur- und Formsehens in Zeichnung und Malerei. In H.H. Wieck (ed.), *Psychopathologie musische Gestaltungen.* Stuttgart: Schattauer, 29–88.

Jung, R. 1984: Electrophysiological cues of the language-dominant hemisphere in man: slow brain potentials during language processing and writing. *Experimental Brain Research*, Suppl. 9, 430–50.

Jung, R. 1985: Cerebral correlates of motor programming and the processing of words and numbers. *Experimental Brain Research*, 58, A14–15.

Kennedy, C., Des Rosiers, M.H., Sakurada, O., Shinohara, M., Reivich, M., Jehle, J.W. and Sokoloff, L. 1976: Metabolic mapping of the primary visual system of the monkey by means of the autoradiographic [^{14}C]deoxyglucose technique. *Proceedings of the National Academy of Science USA, Neurobiology*, 73, 4230–4.

Kohonen, T., Oja, E. and Lehtiö, P. 1981: Storage and processing of information in distributed associative memory systems. In G.E. Hinton and J.A. Anderson (eds), *Parallel Models of Associative Memory.* Hillsdale, NJ: Lawrence Erlbaum Associates.

Kornhuber, H.H. and Deecke, L. 1965: Hirnpotentialänderungen bei Wilkürbewegungen und passiven Bewegungen des Menschen: Bereitschaftspotential und reafferente Potentiale. *Pflügers Archiv für die gesamte Physiologie*, 284, 1–17.

Lashley, K.S. 1950: In search of the engram. Society for Experimental Biology, Symposium no. 4. *Physiological Mechanisms in Animal Behaviour*, 454–82.

Lettvin, J., Maturana, H.R., Pitts, W.H. and McCulloch, W.S. 1959: What the frog's eye tells the frog's brain. *Proceedings of the Institute of Radio Engineers, NY*, 47, 1940–51.

Lynch, G. 1986: *Synapses, Circuits and the Beginnings of Memory*. Cambridge, MA and London: MIT Press.

McCollough, C. 1965: Color adaptation of edge-detectors in the human visual system. *Science*, 149, 1115–16.

MacKay, D.M. 1949: On the combination of digital and analogue techniques in the design of analytical engines. Reprinted as appendix in *The Mechanisation of Thought Processes* (NPL Symp. no. 10, 1958). London: HMSO, 53–65.

MacKay, D.M. 1951: Mindlike behaviour in artefacts. *British Journal for the Philosophy of Science*, 2, 105–21.

MacKay, D.M. 1953: Mindlike behaviour in artefacts (reply to correspondents). *British Journal for the Philosophy of Science*, 3, 352–3.

MacKay, D.M. 1954: Operational aspects of some fundamental concepts of communication. *Synthese*, 9, 182–98.

MacKay, D.M. 1956: Towards an information-flow model of human behaviour. *British Journal of Psychology*, 67, 30–43.

MacKay, D.M. 1958: Perceptual stability of a stroboscopically lit visual field containing self-luminous objects. *Nature*, 181, 507–8.

MacKay, D.M. 1959: Operational aspects of intellect. In *The Mechanisation of Thought Processes* (NPL Symp. no. 10, 1958). London: HMSO, 37–73. Also in H. Billing (ed.) 1961: *Information and Learning*. Munich: Oldenburg.

MacKay, D.M. 1960a: On the logical indeterminacy of a free choice. *Mind*, 69, 31–40.

MacKay, D.M. 1960b: Modelling of large-scale nervous activity. In J.W. Beament (ed.), *Models and Analogues for Biology*. Symposia of the Society for Experimental Biology, 14. London: Cambridge University Press, 192–8. (American edition, New York: Academic Press, 1960.)

MacKay, D.M. 1961: Information and learning. In H. Billing (ed.), *Learning Automata*. Munich: Oldenburg, 40–9.

MacKay, D.M. 1962: Theoretical models of space perception. In C.A. Muses (ed.), *Aspects of the Theory of Artificial Intelligence*. New York: Plenum Press, 83–103.

MacKay, D.M. 1963: Psychophysics of perceived intensity: a theoretical basis for Fechner's and Stevens's laws. *Science*, 139, 1213–16.

MacKay, D.M. 1965a: A mind's eye view of the brain. In Norbert Wiener and J.P. Schadé (eds), *Cybernetics of the Nervous System*, Progress in Brain Research vol. 17. Amsterdam: Elsevier, 321–32.

MacKay, D.M. 1965b: Information and prediction in human sciences. In S. Dockx and P. Bernays (eds), *Information and Prediction in Science*. New York: Academic Press, 255–69.

MacKay, D.M. 1965c: Visual noise as a tool of research. *Journal of General Psychology*, 72, 181–97.

MacKay, D.M. 1966: Conscious control of action. In J.C. Eccles (ed.), *Brain and Conscious Experience*. Heidelberg, New York, Berlin: Springer-Verlag, 422–45.

MacKay, D.M. 1967: The mechanisation of normative behaviour. In L. Thayer (ed.), *Communication Theory and Research*. Springfield, IL: Charles C. Thomas, 228–45.

MacKay, D.M. 1968a: Possible information processing functions of inhibitory mechanisms. In *Structure and Functions of Neuronal Mechanisms*, Proceedings of the Fourth International Meeting of Neurobiologists, Stockholm, September 1966. Oxford and New York: Pergamon.

MacKay, D.M. 1968b: The importance of landmarks in visual perception. In E.R. Caianiello (ed.), *Neural Networks*, Berlin, Heidelberg, New York: Springer-Verlag, 59–64.

MacKay, D.M. 1969: *Information, Mechanism and Meaning*. (Volume I, Selected Papers.) Boston: MIT Press.

MacKay, D.M. 1970: Digits and analogues. In H.E. von Gierke, W.D. Keidel and H.L. Oestreicher (eds), *Principles and Practice of Bionics*. London: Technivision, 457–66.

MacKay, D.M. 1971: The human touch. In O.J. Grüsser and R. Klinke (eds), *Pattern Recognition in Biological and Technical Systems*. Berlin, Heidelberg, New York: Springer-Verlag.

MacKay, D.M. 1972: Formal analysis of communicative processes. In R.A. Hinde (ed.), *Non-verbal Communication*. London: Cambridge University Press.

MacKay, D.M. 1973a: Neurophysiological aspects of vision. In M. Marois (ed.), *From Theoretical Physics to Biology*. Basel: S. Karger, 322–7.

MacKay, D.M. 1973b: Visual stability and voluntary eye movements. In R. Jung (ed.), *The Handbook of Sensory Physiology, Vol. VII/3A*. New York, Heidelberg, Berlin: Springer-Verlag, 307–31.

MacKay, D.M. 1978: *Science, Chance and Providence*. Oxford: Oxford University Press, 59–67.

MacKay, D.M. 1980: *Brains, Machines and Persons*. London: Collins; Grand Rapids, MI: Eerdmans.

MacKay, D.M. 1981: What kind of neural image? *Freiburger Universitätsblätter*, 74, 67–72.

MacKay, D.M. 1982a: Ourselves and our brains: duality without Dualism. *Psychendochrinology*, 7, 285–94.

MacKay, D.M. 1982b: Anomalous perception of extrafoveal motion. *Perception*, 11, 359–60.

MacKay, D.M. 1983: On line source density computation with a minimum of electrodes. *Electroencephalography and Clinical Neurophysiology*, 56, 696–8.

MacKay, D.M. 1984a: Source-density mapping of human visual receptive fields using scalp electrodes. *Experimental Brain Research*, 54, 579–81.

MacKay, D.M. 1984b: Mind talk and brain talk. In M.S. Gazzaniga (ed.), *Handbook of Cognitive Neuroscience*. New York: Plenum, 293–317.

MacKay, D.M. 1985a: Machines, brains and persons. *Zygon*, 20, 401–12.

MacKay, D.M. 1985b: The significance of 'feature sensitivity'. In D. Rose and V.G. Dobson (eds), *Models of the Visual Cortex*, Chichester–New York–Brisbane–Toronto–Singapore: John Wiley and Sons Ltd, 47–53.

MacKay, D.M. 1987: Seeing with moving eyes. In R.L. Gregory (ed.), *The Oxford Companion to the Mind*. Oxford: Oxford University Press.

MacKay, D.M. 1988: *The Open Mind*. London: InterVarsity Press, 191–6.

MacKay, D.M. and MacKay, V. 1975: What causes decay of pattern-contingent chromatic aftereffects? *Vision Research*, 15, 462–4.

MacKay, D.M. and MacKay, V. 1982: Explicit dialogue between left and right half-systems of split brains. *Nature*, 295, 690–1.

MacKay, D.M., MacKay, V. and Rulon, M.J. 1986: Scalp topography of ERP source-densities during visually guided target practice. *Experimental Brain Research*, 64, 434–50.

Martin, K.A.C. 1988: From single cells to simple circuits in the cerebral cortex. *Quarterly Journal of Experimental Physiology*, 73, 637–702.

Martin, K.A.C. and Whitteridge, D. 1984: Form, function, and intracortical projections of spiny neurones in the striate visual cortex of the cat. *Journal of Physiology*, 353, 463–504.

Maxwell, J.C. 1868: On governors. *Proceedings of the Royal Society, London*, 16, 270–83.

Monod, J. 1972: *Chance and Necessity*. London: Collins.

Parfit, D. 1984, *Reasons and Persons*. Oxford: Clarendon.

Peirce, C.S. 1931–58: *Collected Papers of Charles Sanders Peirce*. Cambridge, MA: Harvard University Press.

Penfield, W. 1966: Speech, perception and the uncommitted cortex. In J.C. Eccles (ed.), *Brain and Conscious Experience*. Heidelberg, New York, Berlin: Springer-Verlag, 217–37.

Penfield, W. and Rasmussen, T. 1957: *A Clinical Study of Localization of Function*. New York: Macmillan.

Penfield, W. and Roberts, L. 1959: *Speech and Brain Mechanisms*. Princeton University Press.

Phelps, M.E. and Mazziotta, J.C. 1985: Positron emission tomography: human brain function and biochemistry. *Science*, 228, 799–809.

Phillips, C.G., Zeki, S. and Barlow, H.B. 1984: Localization of function in the cerebral cortex, *Brain*, 107, 327–61.

Polanyi, M. 1967: *The Tacit Dimension*. London: Routledge and Kegan Paul.

Polanyi, M. 1969: *Knowing and Being*. London: Routledge and Kegan Paul.

Popper, K.R. 1950: Indeterminism in quantum physics and in classical physics. *British Journal for the Philosophy of Science*, 1, 117–33; 173–95.

Popper, K.R. and Eccles, J.C. 1977: *The Self and its Brain – an Argument for Interactionism*. Berlin: Springer International.

Porter, P.B. 1954: Another puzzle-picture. *American Journal of Psychology*, 67, 550–1.

Potter, M.C. 1954: Meaning in visual search. *Science*, 187, 965–6.

Price, J.L. and Slotnick, B.M. 1983: Dual olfactory representation in the rat thalamus: an anatomical and electrophysiological study. *Journal of Comparative Neurology*, 215, 63–77.

Puccetti, R. 1973: Brain bisection and personal identity. *British Journal for the Philosophy of Science*, 24, 339–55.

Regan, D. 1968a: Evoked potentials and sensation. *Perception and Psychophysics*, 4, 347–50.

Regan, D. 1968b: A high frequency mechanism which underlies visual evoked potentials. *Electroencephalography and Clinical Neurophysiology*, 25, 231–7.

Reichardt, W. 1957: Autokorrelations-Auswertung als Functionsprinzip des Neuralsystems. *Zeitschrift für Naturforschung*, 12b, 447–57.

Reichardt, W. and Poggio, T. 1976: Visual control of orientation behaviour in the fly. *Quarterly Review of Biophysics*, 9, 311–75.

Reid, T. 1815: From The Works of Thomas Reid. In G. Dworkin (ed.), 1970. *Determinism, Freewill and Moral Responsibility*. Englewood Cliffs, NJ: Prentice-Hall, 92.

Ross, E.D. 1984: Right hemisphere's role in language, affective behaviour and emotion. *Trends in Neurosciences*, 7, 342–6.

Searle, J.R. 1984: *The Reith Lectures: Minds, Brains and Science*. London: British Broadcasting Corporation.

Segundo, P. 1970: Communication and coding by nerve cells. In F.O. Schmitt (ed.), *The Neurosciences: Second Study Program*. New York: Rockerfeller University Press.

Sholl, D.A. 1956: *The Organisation of the Cerebral Cortex*. London: Methuen.

Sokoloff, L. 1977: Relation between physiological function and energy metabolism in the central nervous system. *Journal of Neurochemistry*, 29, 13–26.

Sokoloff, L., Reivich, M., Kennedy, C., Des Rosiers, M.H., Patlak, C.S., Pettigrew, K.D., Sakurada, O. and Shinohara, M. 1977: The [¹⁴C]deoxy-glucose method for the measurement of local cerebral glucose utilization: theory, procedure, and normal values in the conscious and anesthetized albino rat. *Journal of Neurochemistry*, 28, 897–916.

Somogyi, P., Kisvárday, Z.F., Martin, K.A.C. and Whitteridge, D. 1983: Synaptic connections of morphologically identified and physiologically characterised large basket cells in the striate cortex of the cat. *Neuro-science*, 10, 261–94.

Sperry, R.W. 1968: Hemisphere deconnection and unity in conscious aware-ness. *American Psychologist*, 23, 723–33.

Sperry, R.W. 1980: Mind–brain interaction: mentalism, yes; dualism, no. *Neuroscience*, 5, 195–206.

Sperry, R.W. 1983: *Science and Moral Priority*. Oxford: Basil Blackwell.

Stevens, S.S. 1957: On the psychological law. *Psychological Review*, 64, 153–81.

Stevens, S.S. 1961: To honor Fechner and repeal his law. *Science*, 133, 80–6.

Stevens, S.S. 1962: The surprising simplicity of sensory metrics. *American Psychologist*, 17, 29–39.

Swinburne, R.G. 1986: *The Evolution of the Soul*. Oxford: Clarendon Press.

Teuber, H.-L., Battersby, W.S. and Bender, M.B. 1960: *Visual Field Defects after Penetrating Missile Wounds of the Brain*. Cambridge, MA: Harvard University Press.

Thomson, Sir William 1881: The tide gauge, tidal harmonic analyser and tide predicter. *Proceedings of the Institute of Civil Engineers*, 65, 2–25.

Turing, A.M. 1937: On computable numbers with an application to the Endscheidungs-Problem. *Proceedings of the London Mathematical Society (2)*, 42, 230–65.

Turing, A.M. 1950: Computing machinery and intelligence. *Mind*, 59, 433–60.

Valla, L. translated 1970: Dialogue on free will. In G. Dworkin (ed.), *Determinism, Freewill and Moral Responsibility*. Englewood Cliffs, NJ: Pren-tice-Hall, 115.

Vickers, Sir Geoffrey 1964: The psychology of policy making and social change. *British Journal of Psychiatry*, 110, 465–77.

Vickers, Sir Geoffrey 1965: *The Art of Judgment, a Study of Policy Making*. London: Chapman and Hall.

Watson, J.B. 1930: *Behaviorism*, 2nd edn. London: Kegal Paul, Trench and Trubner.

Wittgenstein, L. 1922: *Tractatus Logico-Philosophicus*. London: Kegan Paul, Trench and Trubner, proposition 6.522.

Zeki, S.M. 1978: Functional specialisation in the visual cortex of the rhesus monkey. *Nature*, 274, 423–8.

Zeki, S.M. 1984: The specialization of function and the function of specialization in the visual cortex. In P.F. Baker (ed.), *Recent Advances in Physiology, 10*. Edinburgh: Churchill Livingstone, 67–85.

Index